Computers and Clinical Audit

Computers and Clinical Audit

AN INTRODUCTION FOR DOCTORS AND HEALTH
CARE PROFESSIONALS

Sue Kinn

Research Fellow
Glasgow University
Scotland

and

Tanya Siann

Audit Co-ordinator
Lanarkshire Health Board
Scotland

SPRINGER-SCIENCE+BUSINESS MEDIA, B.V.

First edition 1993

© 1993 Sue Kinn and Tanya Siann
Originally published by Chapmann & Hall in 1993

Typeset in 10/12 Times by EXPO Holdings, Malaysia

ISBN 978-0-412-49280-8   ISBN 978-1-4899-6639-1 (eBook)
DOI 10.1007/978-1-4899-6639-1

A catalogue record for this book is available from the British Library

Library of Congress Cataloging-in-Publication data available

∞ Printed on permanent acid-free text paper, manufactured in accordance with
ANSI/NISO Z 39.48 – 1992 and ANSI Z 39.48 – 1984

Contents

Preface

There are many books on audit in general, or audit within specific specialties. There are very few books that contain much practical information about computers and their use in audit. Those that exist tend to look at computerised audit systems which are already available and which can be customised for use with individual projects.

Our experience of training health care professionals has shown us that there is a great demand for basic, practical information, which can be used to make informed choices about the types of computer systems required for audit. Most of this information is available but in very disparate places. Having spent many hours collecting it together for ourselves we decided to gather it together into one book. We have tried to make the book as free from jargon and as readable as possible. In particular we have included a glossary of terms which may be useful when reading other articles or books about computers. We hope that this book will help you make informed decisions about your use of computers and we would welcome any comments about the material we have covered.

We have tried to avoid mentioning any application packages or computerised audit systems by name, although in some cases it has been unavoidable. Computer technology is changing so rapidly that any such information could be outdated by the time the book is published. We hope that this book will give you the necessary understanding to be able to refer to the numerous regular computer magazines, available at any newsagent, which provide a good source of comprehensive and up-to-date information on the latest computer developments.

We recommend, if you are considering buying any equipment, that you consult the computer magazines and any technically minded people to whom you have access for advice about both hardware and software.

The content of the book was divided so that Chapters 1,3,4,5,6,7 and 8 were written by Sue Kinn and Chapters 2,9,11 and 12 were written by Tanya Siann; Chapter 10 was a joint effort. We hope that this explains any perceived differences in style between different parts of the book.

The following terms have been used throughout the text; they are the names of some of the companies that manufacture hardware and software, or the names of specific types of software. They are registered trademarks: Microsoft, Microsoft Windows, Unix, IBM, Apple Macintosh, Amstrad, Digital Research, Pick, VME, VM/IS, BOS, DOS, Intel, Lotus, Motorola, DEC, OS/2, Sinclair Spectrum, Atari, BBC computers.

Special thanks are due to Jacqueline Riordan and Iona Young who helped with the preparation of some of the manuscript.

Finally, we would like to thank our friends and families for putting up with our absences while we were writing the book.

PART ONE
Introduction to Computers

Part One will concentrate on introducing the reader to the computer and unravelling the mysteries associated with it. The contents of each chapter are outlined below.

Chapter 1 Covers the different parts of the computer (or hardware) and how they fit together. It also explains some of the jargon associated with computers.

Chapter 2 Covers the history of the computer and the development of the PC in detail.

Chapter 3 Introduces operating systems, specifically DOS, the Disk Operating System, which is the most common operating system for PCs.

Chapter 4 Discusses the range of software, or application packages that are available.

Chapter 5 Looks at the principles of database design.

Chapter 6 Covers the extracting of data from databases.

Chapter 7 Looks at the the concepts of spreadsheets.

Chapter 8 Introduces the concepts of word processors.

Chapter 9 Discusses the principles involved in sharing data between different application packages and different users.

The order in which the chapters about the different application packages are presented reflects their importance for audit.

Introduction to the hardware | 1

Hardware has been defined as: 'the parts of the computer that make a noise when you become so frustrated that you throw them on the floor!'

Modern computer hardware is very varied and the choices available for the computer novice can be overwhelming. Most of the problems that people have with computers stem from a lack of understanding of the jargon. Like all subjects the simple can be made very complicated by cloaking it with mysterious words. This chapter will explain what the different bits of the hardware are, how they fit together and some of the terms which are used to describe them.

This chapter will give you an introduction to the different types of hardware devices available. It has been arranged to describe the components of the basic *IBM-compatible personal computer (PC)* as you might unpack it from a box. It then goes on to describe other hardware devices that you may encounter. The discussion, although based on the PC, is relevant to all computers.

Introducing the personal computer

A computer is a device which will allow large amounts of data to be processed and manipulated at high speed. This data can be numeric, graphic, textual, video, or a mixture of all of these. The basic component of a computer is silicon. At the heart of a computer are lots of circuits etched out on silicon chips; these chips need not concern users at all. It is the type of software package you are working with which will determine what type of data you can use and this is the subject of subsequent chapters. There are certain features that are common to all computers: these are shown in Figure 1.1.

With any computer there has to be some form of *input* so that you can get your data or instructions into the computer. So that you know if the computer has performed as requested there is some form of *output*. All of the processing happens in the *central processing unit (CPU)*. The *memory* of the computer is

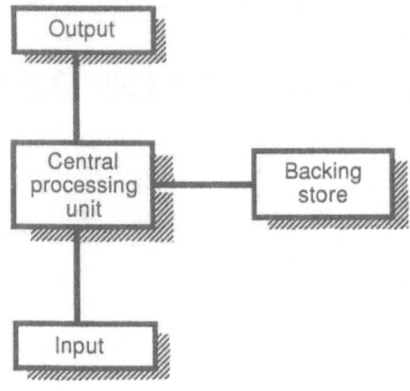

Figure 1.1 The basic structure of the computer.

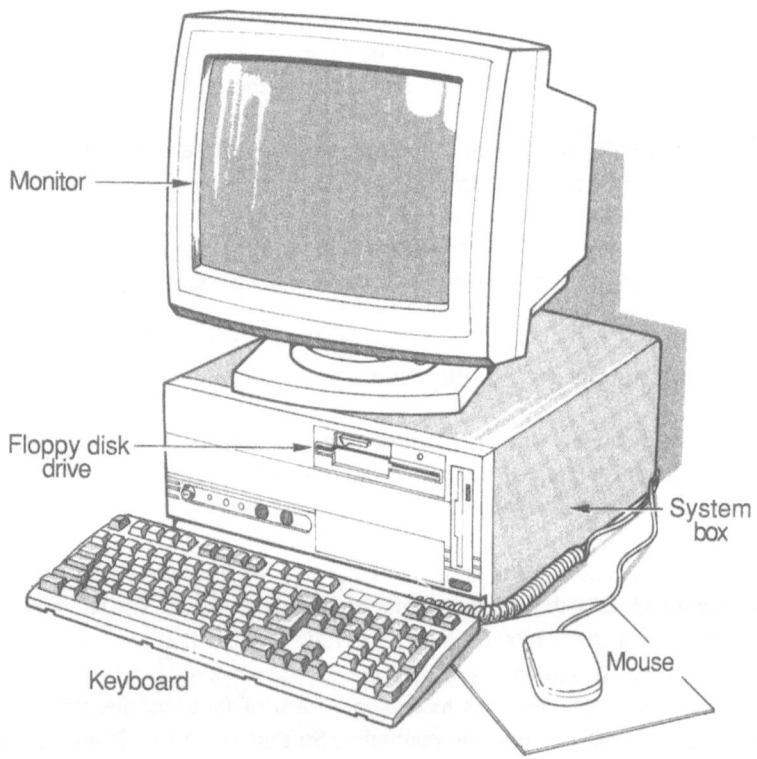

Figure 1.2 The typical personal computer.

part of the CPU. The memory is limited in size, and generally holds information as long as the power to the computer is switched on (p. 15). So that there is a facility to store data and look at it again at some later date there is a need for *backing store*. You can certainly learn how to use a computer without knowing anything about what is going on inside. The next section will cover these different parts of a personal computer (PC) as you might unpack it from a box. After that there will be a brief discussion of other input, output and storage devices that you may have come across in more specialist capacities.

Figure 1.2 shows a typical PC with the different components labelled. The *input* devices shown are the *keyboard* and *mouse*. The *disk drives* can also act as input devices. The output device is the *monitor* or *VDU*. The backing store comprises the disk drives (both the *hard disk* and *floppy disks*). The central processing unit is inside the *system box*. It is a *microprocessor* or *chip*, embedded in the complex circuitry.

Input devices

The keyboard

This is probably the most common form of input into a computer at the present time. The computer keyboard is very much like a typewriter keyboard with extra keys added. There are two types of keyboard available, *normal* or *enhanced* keyboards. Figure 1.3 shows the layout of an enhanced keyboard.

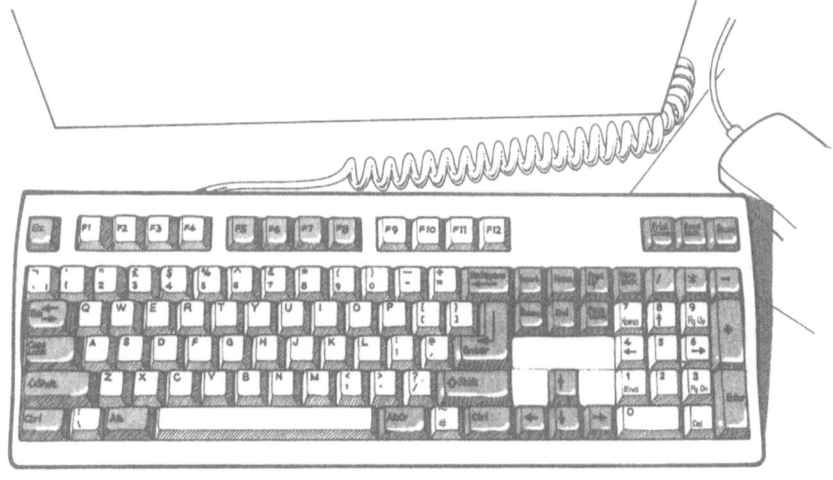

Figure 1.3 The enhanced keyboard.

Normal and enhanced keyboards Normal keyboards are generally found on older computers and on small, compact, portable computers. The difference between a normal and an enhanced keyboard is in the number of keys on the keyboard; normal keyboards have fewer keys. Normal and enhanced keyboards have a number pad, generally to the right of the keyboard. The number keys are arranged like a calculator. However each key has a number and sometimes a word or an arrow printed on it as well. It is very useful to be able to have all the numbers grouped together to enter numeric data: it saves you having to pick the numbers out from across the top of the keyboard. Sometimes you will want to use the arrow keys, which are also referred to as cursor keys, to move around the screen or the word keys which perform certain functions in software packages. To switch between the number function of the key and the arrow, or word, function of the key can be time consuming, and introduce errors. Enhanced keyboards have got round this switching problem by duplicating the arrows and words into separate key pads, so that they appear twice on the keyboard. This means that you can use a number pad to enter numbers and the arrow keys or cursor pad to move around the screen.

Another difference between normal and enhanced keyboards is the number of *function keys*. Function keys are grouped across the top, or down the left hand side of the keyboard. They are labelled from F1 to F10 or F12. There are ten function keys on a normal keyboard and twelve function keys on an enhanced keyboard. Function keys are often used as a quick way of giving instructions to the computer. Pressing F1 will generally instruct the machine to display any available *Help* in most software packages. If you get to a point where you are stuck using a piece of software and want help on the subject, rather than having to go back to the manual and finding out where the Help is, pressing F1 will give Help instructions on the screen. The rest of the function keys are generally assigned to software-specific functions. You will have to get used to the function keys in the particular software packages that you are using. The rest of the keyboard, the QWERTY, or letter, part of the keyboard, is very much like the standard typewriter keyboard.

Extra keys on the keyboard Computers also have some important extra keys. The first key to note is the Escape key, often abbreviated to ESC. This can be very useful if you get to a point where you are using a piece of software where nothing seems to be happening, you appear to be locked, or you find that you are lost within the software and cannot recognise what to do next. Pressing the Escape key can sometimes release you from that lock, or that unfamiliar area. If you press ESC several times you may find that you actually go back several stages to a point that you recognise and can move forward from. This saves you having to turn the machine off and then back on again. Escape does not always work, but it is certainly a useful key to try first.

The next keys to note are those labelled CTRL for Control and ALT for Alternate. These are ways of giving the computer shorthand instructions. The letter A on the keyboard is used in any text you may be entering; however CTRL and A or ALT and A may be shorthand ways of telling the computer to do a particular instruction. These keys effectively increase the different key combinations available to give instructions to the computer. As you become more expert in using your computer system, you will recognise that this can save you a lot of time. CTRL and ALT work very much like the Shift key. In a standard typewriter, and indeed a computer, if you wish to get a capital letter, or the uppermost character where there is more than one character on the key, you press the Shift key. There is a Shift key on either side of the letter part of the keyboard (they have large, upward facing, open arrows and sometimes the word SHIFT). While you keep the Shift key depressed you then press the key which you are interested in. To get a capital A, for instance, you press SHIFT, keeping your finger on the Shift key and press A at the same time, then release both of the keys simultaneously. This will give you a capital A as opposed to a lower case a. CTRL and ALT work similarly. You press and hold either CTRL or ALT and then the relevant key, and then release both of them at the same time.

At the right hand side of the letter keyboard is a key labelled BACKSPACE; this has a backward facing filled in black arrow. If you type the wrong character which you then want to remove you simply press this key. It will delete the immediately preceding character. It deletes from left to right across the screen. Press it three times: it will delete the last three characters you typed in. Unlike the backspace key on a typewriter, you do not use this key to move back along a line you have already typed. For this you use the cursor keys. The Delete key (DEL) is found on the number pad and the word pad on the enhanced keyboard. This will remove characters to the right of the cursor within some software packages. The *cursor* is the mark that indicates the position you are typing in from (Chapter 3). Underneath the Backspace key is an ENTER or RETURN key; this sometimes has a bent arrow drawn on it and is labelled by the word ENTER (sometimes RETURN). This is like a carriage return on a typewriter. Press this key if you want to start a new line. When you are using the computer you have to indicate that you wish the computer to execute (perform) a command and pressing the ENTER key is the way to do this.

Along the bottom of the keyboard is a larger key called the Spacebar. As with a typewriter, you press this bar if you wish to make a space between characters. Unlike a typewriter, you do not use this key to move forward along a line you have already typed. For this you use the cursor keys.

Mouse

The *mouse* is an electronic pointing device. If you use a piece of software which supports a mouse, there will be some form of pointer on the screen. This may be an arrow, cross or some other shape. As you move the mouse across the top of the desk the pointer on the screen will also move. As you move the mouse up, the pointer moves up. If you move the mouse to the right, the pointer will move to the right and so on. Underneath the mouse is a small ball which moves as you move the mouse. The pointer on the screen is linked to the movements of this ball.

You indicate to the machine, or *activate*, any item that you are interested in by pointing at it and clicking one of the mouse buttons. Most mice have two buttons, some have three. Generally the leftmost mouse button is the one which is used most often. The right hand button is really there to allow for an expansion of possible tasks in the future.

The mouse is a very intuitive way of using the computer and has certainly achieved a great degree of success with computers like the Apple Macintosh. There has been an increase in graphical software, that produces pictures on the screen. The use of mice has increased with these developments and is discussed elsewhere (Chapter 4).

Output devices

Visual display unit (VDU)

The most common form of output is the *visual display unit* (VDU). Sometimes this is also called the *visual display terminal* (VDT) or monitor. While you are using the computer you will be looking at the screen, to measure your progress or to see the result of the last command that you issued. There are many different types of display now available. The most common are based on cathode ray tubes, like those used in televisions. The smaller, portable computers use liquid crystal display (LCD) screens or gas plasma displays.

LCD screens are light and use little power. This means that they are ideal for portable, battery operated machines. They show dark characters on a lighter background. They do not show contrast well and the response time is quite slow. This means that the screen can appear blurred if an image moves across it rapidly.

Colour screens are becoming more popular for laptop computers. There are two types at present, active and passive matrices. Active matrices, which are more expensive, give the best quality image and are able to display more colours than the passive matrices.

Gas plasma screens need mains power. They show text as orange on a dark orange background. They do not show contrast too well. They are sometimes used in laptop machines that are made to be transported around, but not used away from a mains power source.

The cathode ray tube monitors can be monochrome or colour. The monitor performance is often measured in resolution – the number of pixels, or picture elements. This is quoted as, for example, 640 by 400. This means 640 pixels across and 400 down the screen. The more pixels, the better the resolution of the screen.

There are different types of display or screens that you may come across. The earliest were the monochrome Hercules screens, which could only display one colour. The earliest of the colour screens was the CGA (Colour Graphics Array).

These have low resolution and for text letters can be difficult to distinguish. A later development is the EGA (Enhanced Graphics Array). This has a better resolution with good graphics and text. The standard today is VGA (Video Graphics Array). This has better resolution and has excellent graphics and text display. SVGA (Super VGA) is a further refinement.

The VGA output is to an analogue monitor. Analogue monitors can show a vast range of brightness for each colour. This is one of the reasons that the VGA display is superior to the other types. The CGA and EGA output both use digital monitors: that means they can show only two brightness levels for each colour – either On or Off.

For a monitor to work there has to be a *video card* plugged into the computer, within the system box. The card can then direct the output to the monitor, in the appropriate form. The actual function of the card need not concern most users but it is important to make sure that you have the correct card in place if you are changing your VDU at any time.

Monitors are based on cathode ray tubes and they have a light-sensitive layer on the inside of the screen. If the same image is projected onto the screen for any length of time it can be etched into this layer. This means that you will be able to see this image, even if the machine is switched off. To prevent this from happening it is always a good idea to turn the screen off if you are not going to be looking at it for a period of 30 minutes or so. Some computers have an automatic switch that turns off the screen, after a predetermined time interval, if no key presses are registered. Pressing any key will cause the screen display to reappear. There are also some programs, called screen savers, that can be installed on the machine. If the screen display does not change, after a predetermined time the *screen saver* becomes active. It may be moving patterns, fish swimming in a tank, or a variety of other pictures. As they are constantly moving, they prevent the inside of the screen from being damaged.

Other output devices, such as printers, are discussed on p. 16.

Backing store

If you have been working on the computer and wish to save your data you have to save it to the *backing store*. Storage usually takes the form of disks, although magnetic tape is also used. For the IBM compatible PC, which has become fairly standard in the National Health Service, the backing storage devices commonly used are hard and floppy disks. The floppy disk is a magnetic disk in a plastic protective cover. A hard disk, inside the system box, is like a record or stack of records. They are both discussed in more detail below.

Hard disks

Hard disks are sited within the system box of the computer. Data is read from or written to the disk by means of disk heads. These can be likened to the arms and

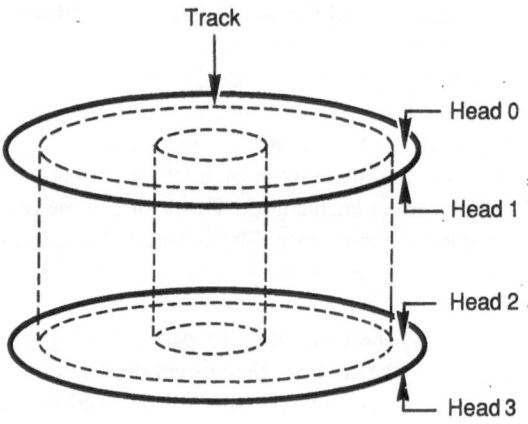

Figure 1.4 The arrangement of disks within a hard disk unit.

needles of a record player. The arms can move and position the heads on the appropriate part of the disk. Hard disks are like a stack of records one on top of the other. Each side of each hard disk has got its own needle, known as a *read/write head* (Figure 1.4).

If you request information from the hard disk, the stack of disks will rotate. The heads will move in and out along the disk. When one head finds the information the stack stops rotating. The information can then be read from the disk. The movement of all of the read/write heads is synchronised, so that they all move in and out along the surface of the disk together. The disks are actually quite delicate and when the machine has to be moved the heads sometimes have to be *parked*. This is like securing the needle on a record player. In some machines this is done automatically and you do not have to worry about it, but in others you actually have to give a command to do this. If you do need to use this command it is a good idea always to do so before switching off the computer.

Capacity of hard disks A hard disk is divided up into tracks. These are concentric circles which start at the outside and move to the inside of the disk. They are discrete circles and are actually not visible if you look at the surface of a hard disk. They are formed by the arrangement of the magnetic particles on the disk. The tracks are divided up into sectors, like slices of a cake. Figure 1.5 shows a bird's-eye view of the surface of a disk. The number of tracks and sectors will depend on the type of disk. Generally the manual of the computer will give you information about your hard disk and its capacity. There will be some information somewhere about how many bytes of information each sector holds, how many sectors there are per track, how many tracks per side and how many sides on the disk. This will then be multiplied together to give you the capacity of your hard disk. So what is a byte?

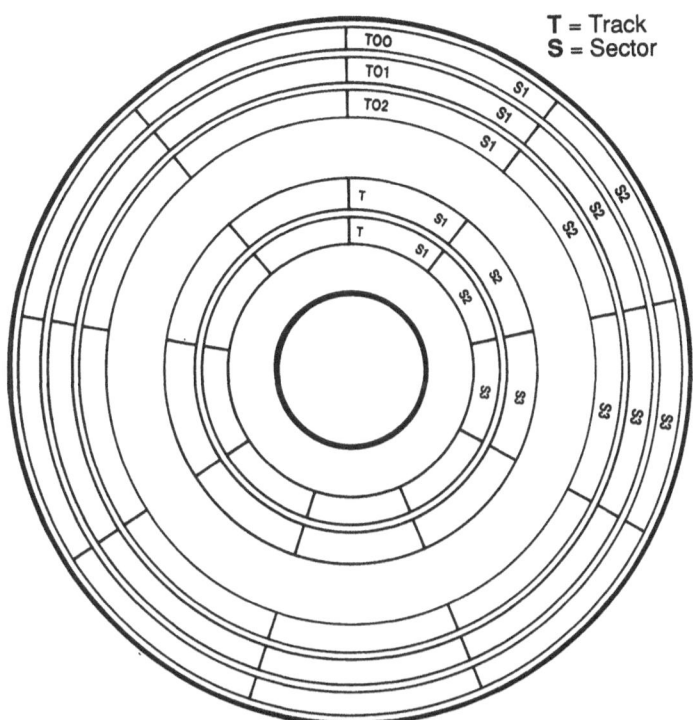

Figure 1.5 A bird's eye view of the tracks and sectors on both hard and floppy disks. The number of tracks and sectors will vary depending on the type of disk.

Bytes Computers store all information as a series of binary digits. The words *binary digit* are abbreviated to form the word *bit*. Each bit is either a 1 or a 0. These bits are then grouped together in collections of eight. These eight bits are called a *byte*. So eight bits is one byte. The reason to collect them together in groups of eight is that this gives you many different unique possibilities. If there are eight 1 and 0s in a line there are 256 unique combinations. There are enough combinations to represent every character on the keyboard, the letters A–Z in upper and lower case, all the numbers and all the other characters and still have some combinations available for control characters. When the computer beeps at you while you are using it, the information for that beep is held as one byte. If you press the space bar this is also stored as one byte, a combination of eight 1s and 0s.

If your manual states that each sector holds 256 bytes this means that each sector can hold 256 characters. By working out the multiplication of bytes x sectors x tracks x sides you can work out the capacity of the hard disk. This will probably be something over 40 million bytes, known as 40 megabytes. One *megabyte* (Mb) is a million bytes. Sometimes you will see storage (or memory) referred to in terms of kilobytes. One *kilobyte* (Kb) is a thousand bytes.

Floppy disks

There are different types of floppy disks. There are the larger 5¼ inch and the smaller 3½ inch disks. Some computers will have a floppy disk drive for one size or the other; occasionally computers have disk drives for the two different disk sizes.

The 5¼" disks, the larger of the floppy disk sizes, are quite flimsy. If you touch them they bend fairly easily. They slide into the disk drive. There is a gate on the drive. Shut the gate by rotating it through 90°; the disk is then ready to be used. To remove the disk the gate has to be opened.

The 3½" disks are much more sturdy. They do not appear to bend when pressed or touched. They have a metal cover at one end. These disks are slotted into the disk drive. The disk drive will have a small button by the side of it. Once the disk is in place the button pops out. To remove the disk you simply press this button and the disk is ejected.

Both types of drive have lights on them. The lights illuminate if the computer is either reading from or writing to the disk. There is a similar light to indicate if information is being read from or written to the hard disk.

Inside the covers of both types of disks there is a floppy magnetic disk. The surface is shiny grey. Both types look the same, except for the obvious size difference. This is the actual floppy disk. The plastic covering on the outside is for protection. In both types of disk there is a sector cut out of the cover. Once inserted into the disk drive the disk rotates within its protective covering. This allows the whole surface of the disk to be examined by the read/write heads, through the cut out sector of the cover.

In the larger 5¼" disk the sector is cut out of the protective cover and you can see the surface of the disk beneath. When you insert the disk into the disk drive the read/write heads for the disk access information from this exposed portion of the disk. For the smaller 3½" disk, as you insert the disk into the disk drive the metal cover at the top of the disk moves to one side. You can actually slide this back yourself and can see that there is actually a cut out plastic sector visible underneath the metal. The smaller 3½" disks offer disks more protection, as they are in a more sturdy robust cover and the cut out sector is covered by the metal sheath the majority of the time. These disks, which are more expensive, are much easier to transport around and send to other people.

Double density and high density disks There are actually two different types of each disk size. There are *double density (DD)* and *high density (HD) disks*. If you look at a bird's-eye view of the surface of the disk (and this applies to both sizes), you will see that, like the hard disk, they are divided up into tracks and sectors (Figure 1.5). For double density disks there are 40 tracks and nine sectors. In high density disks there are 80 tracks and 15 sectors. The high density disks are a technological development from the double density disks which were invented first. It is just a refinement which allows more tracks and sectors to be

Table 1.1 The size, density and capacity of the different types of floppy disk

Size	Density	Format	Disk Type	
5¼"	DD	360 Kb	Double sided DD	48 TPI
5¼"	HD	1.2 Mb	Double sided HD	96 TPI
3½"	DD	760 Kb	Double sided DD	135 TPI
3½"	HD	1.4 Mb	Double sided HD	135 TPI

DD, double density; HD, high density; Kb, kilobytes; Mb, megabytes;
TPI, Tracks per inch.

produced on the same area. The number of tracks is determined by the number of magnetic particles which are deposited on the surface of the disks. This does have some important implications. Machines which use double density disks tend to be older, developed before the high density disks were invented. They are unable to read the high density disks. High density machines, however, can read not only high density disks but, because the double density disks were already in existence, they can read them too. If you want to exchange information with colleagues you need to find out not only the size of the disk required, but also the density of the disk.

Table 1.1 gives the size, density and capacity of the different types of disks. You will see that the capacities are unique for the different sizes and the different densities. This is sometimes the easiest way to remember which type of disk you require. If you go into a shop and ask for a 360 K disk, you will automatically be given a 5¼" double density disk. If you ask for a 1.4 Mb disk you will automatically be given a 3½" high density disk and so on.

Write protecting floppy disks If you have information on a disk which you feel is very valuable, and which you want to be sure you will not lose, you can *write protect* your disk. There is an analogy with audio-cassette tapes. If you record something onto the tape that you do not wish to lose you can remove a small tab at the top of the cassette which prevents re-recording. If you cover the resulting notch with some sticky tape you are then able to re-record as normal. Write protecting disks follows the same principle.

With the 5¼" disk there is a small notch cut out of the side of the disk's protective cover. If you are looking at the upper side of the disk you see this notch at the top right hand corner. Cover this notch with an opaque piece of tape or sticky label and you can read any information from the disk, but are unable to write anything to it. When you buy the 5¼" disks you should get some sticky labels for this purpose. If you want to write onto the disk at a later date all you have to do is remove the label from the notch.

With the 3½" disk if you turn it so that the circular metal spindle is uppermost, at the bottom right hand side of the disk is a button which can slide up and down. If you slide the button down you will notice that there is a hole through the disk in this corner. This disk is now write protected and you are unable to write anything onto it. If you decide, at a later date, that you do want to write onto the disk simply slide the button up.

Storing floppy disks Disks are made of magnetic material. The information is stored by the magnetic particles on the disk. If you place a disk beside a strong magnet you can corrupt the data. When you put your disk into the machine again you may find that it is totally unreadable and that you have lost a lot of information. One cause of magnetic disturbance is the telephone. As the telephone rings it creates magnetic fluxes that can corrupt the disk. Do not store your disks any where near telephones or other magnets. Another hazard for disks are the magnetic 'keys' that are used for some cat-flaps. If you use one of these, do not let your cat sit near your disks! Computers generate heat and cats often seek them out so be careful! There are usually warnings about the care of disks on the package.

It is all right to place a disk into a disk drive before you turn on the computer. You may want to do this if you are starting your computer from a system disk (p. 29). Remove disks before you turn the machine off, however: the magnetic surges as you switch off are greater than when turning on and this can corrupt the data.

Formatting floppy disks When you buy floppy disks you are not able to use them straight away as they are not *formatted*. Formatting involves laying down the magnetic tracks and sectors. Once this has been done the read/write heads in the disk drives are able to read from or write to the disks. There is a special operating system command to prepare (or format) the disks for use. This is discussed in Chapter 3.

Central Processing Unit (CPU)

In Figure 1.2 the system box was labelled as containing the *central processing unit*. This is the heart of the computer. It is a microprocessor or chip that is part of the complex circuitry of the computer.

There are a variety of chips available. They are becoming faster and more powerful all the time. Quite often the machine will be referred to according to the type of CPU or chip that it contains. The first PCs used 8088 chips. The next series had 80286 and at present machines are being manufactured using 80386 and 80486 chips. The latest developments are concerned with the 80586 chip which is called the Pentium. These numbers are often abbreviated to 286, 386 and 486. The higher the number the more modern the chip. A good analogy to chip size is car engine size. A car with a 1000cc engine will not perform as well as a similar car with a 2500cc engine.

These chips form a family of microprocessors. Other microprocessors are used in other types of computer. Because the chips form a chronological sequence, software written for an early chip will work on the later versions. However software written for a later version will not work (or not work properly) on earlier versions. The different chips are described in more detail in Chapter 2.

There are three parts to the CPU. These are the *arithmetic logic unit (ALU)*, the *control unit* and the *memory*. The arithmetic logic unit is where all the number crunching and text handling is done. The control unit controls the flow of information into the ALU. If all the numbers you wanted to add up arrived at the ALU at the same time the result at the end would not be reliable. The control unit makes sure that each number is trickled into the ALU one at a time so that each one is included in the sum. Memory will be discussed separately.

Memory

There are two types of memory, the *Read Only Memory (ROM)* and the *Random Access Memory (RAM)*. The memory is located on separate chips from the main processor and communicates with it.

Read Only Memory (ROM) The instructions in ROM allow the computer to begin the start up process (booting up) which will enable the computer to get to a state so that the user can use it. These starting instructions are etched into the chip. They are always present in the computer. Each time you switch on, the computer follows the same instructions. If you want to change these instructions you generally have to take out the ROM chip and replace it with another.

Random Access Memory (RAM) This is sometimes called read and write memory or volatile memory.

RAM serves two functions. First some of the software instructions are held in the memory. This means that they are instantly accessible to the machine. When the machine is booting up some of the commands for the operating system (Chapter 3) are loaded into memory. If you have loaded a word processing package some of its instructions will also be in memory. If you instruct the machine to underline a heading, if the instruction is in memory it will happen instantly. If the instruction is not in memory the machine will have to find it on the disk, read it into memory and then execute the instruction. This will take much longer. The more instructions that can be held in the memory the faster the machine will carry out the task required. The second function of RAM is that it acts as a data reservoir. As you open documents to edit, in your word processor (or database files to process etc.), these are loaded into the memory. The more memory the computer has the more information (instructions and data) it can store. The CPU keeps the instructions and data apart.

If there is a power cut or you turn off the machine the contents of this memory are lost, hence it is known as volatile memory. If you do not save work that you are doing it will be lost when the electricity supply is cut off. You will probably find that you lose some work once through not saving, and that thereafter you save very regularly. By saving every 10 or 15 minutes you can never lose too much work. Some of the more modern software now allows you to set time intervals, after which it prompts, or asks if you want to save your work.

The processor and the memory have to communicate. There are special wires that allow the bits (1s and 0s) to move from memory to processor and vice versa. These wires are collectively known as a bus. A bus is like a motorway: the wider it is the more traffic (or bits) it can carry. As the bus becomes wider the computer becomes faster, more bits can move through the bus in a set period of time. As chips have developed the buses have become wider, moving from 8 lanes to 32 lanes (Chapter 2).

To read information into the memory the computer relies on the backing store, or disks. The backing store is like a library. The information (or instructions and data) is stored until required. It is then read into the memory of the computer. The data can be altered and saved onto the backing store. The next time it is read into the memory it will be in its updated version.

Other hardware devices

The computer has several ports, or plugs, at the back of the system box. This allows you to add extra peripherals (hardware) to the machine. You may decide that you require an extra disk drive, a mouse, a printer, a joy-stick and so on. These can be bought and plugged into the machine at the appropriate port. You will then need appropriate software (instructions) to indicate to the machine that these hardware devices are plugged in and you wish to use them. This type of software is often small programs called *device drivers*. Generally when you buy the peripherals they will come with a floppy disk and instructions about how to install the device driver.

Some of the range of hardware devices available are discussed below, grouped according to whether they relate to Input, Output or the Backing store. Some of the peripherals you may have come across in your working environment, or in public display computers. Occasionally you may wish to use them with your own computer set-up.

Input devices

Punched cards

This is a very old method of input that you are now unlikely to see. The cards had a series of holes punched in them. Each card represented one line of instructions for the computer. As programs have become more and more sophisticated, the number of cards required would be unmanageable. There were many operational problems with cards. If one of the corners got bent, the cards were in the wrong order, or a card got lost the whole computer program would come to a grinding halt.

Touch screen

When you use a touch screen as input, you actually touch the computer screen. Depending on the position that you touch, the computer will branch to show you a particular part of the program. Such screens are becoming increasingly more common in stations and information bureaux where the screen will display either a particular timetable in which you are interested or what's on at the theatre, cinema etc. These special screens usually detect the touch by having infra red light shining across and down the screen. As you put your finger through the infra red light you create an interference pattern. The computer can work out where you touched the screen, and display the appropriate information.

Light pen

A light pen is a pen which you shine at the relevant part of the screen. Software which allows you to use a light pen generally has a large number of boxes displayed on the screen. Just point or shine the pen at the box you are interested in and more information will appear on the screen.

Optical character readers and optical mark readers (OCR and OMR)

Optical character readers and optical mark readers (abbreviated to OCR or OMR) are increasingly sophisticated devices which can read very stylised characters or marks, such as the strange numbers which you find at the bottom of your bank cheques. Optical character readers have been built that read a variety of different type faces and have been combined with voice synthesizers so that blind people can use them to read bills, magazines etc. Optical mark readers are becoming a more common way of inputting information into computers. They have been used extensively with multiple choice question papers which can then be marked using a computer. Some data collection forms are designed so that they can be filled in by putting a stroke through the appropriate box and read rapidly into the computer.

Scanners

Scanners are devices that read text, or graphics, from paper. They scan the paper and reproduce the image as a file on the computer. The technology is still in its infancy. It does not always recognise characters and requires a good quality image to scan from. At present their use is limited. They are useful to scan large documents to prevent retyping, or for getting drawings or graphics into the computer.

Digitisers

These are magnetic pads. Maps, photographs, diagrams etc. can be placed on them. Areas can be marked using special pens and the computer can put in any required details, such as contours etc. They can be used to work out volumes of tumours, from images, to calculate appropriate doses of radiation etc.

Magnetic tape

Very large computer systems store a lot of information on magnetic tape. This can then be input into the computer by reading the tape. It is a very cheap way of storing large amounts of information, but because it is a linear method of inputting information it has its drawbacks. If you are not sure at what point along the tape the information you require is stored, you have to start at the beginning and keep reading until you find it, a bit like searching a cassette tape until you find the track you want to listen to.

Disks

Disks are made of magnetic material and are used to store information that can be input to a computer. They are much faster to use than tape, because the computer can access different areas of the disk randomly without having to play from one end to the other. They are known as *Random Access Storage devices*. A record is a good analogy, if you want to play the seventh track on a record all you have to do is position the needle over the seventh track and it will be played. This is as quick as playing the fifth track. The average time to find any data on a disk is the same, irrespective of where the data is stored.

Bar codes

A bar code is a pattern of black and white strips that represent a number. Using the special bar code reader, which is either run over the bar code strip or shone at the strip, long numbers can be entered into a computer rapidly. The computer can then match up the number that has been input with stored information about it. This has become common in libraries, supermarkets and medical record departments over the past few years. In the supermarket the computer registers your purchase on the cash register and it also takes that item from the stock list. The two functions have been integrated into one.

Speech

Speech input is becoming more refined. There are some computer voice-activated information phone lines where a computer-simulated voice will give you a list of options and by saying 'Yes' at an appropriate time the computer will branch to tell you more information about your chosen subject.

Speech input is beginning to appear in the Health Service. There are some systems where you can talk through a telephone into the computer. These computers have a list of known words. Present technology recognises these words about 70 per cent of the time. As this technology is refined further, it will one day be fairly easy to dictate information straight into the computer.

Output devices

There are a variety of output devices available. The most common, the VDU, has already been discussed above.

Printers

The advent of computer technology was supposed to herald the introduction of the paper-less office, but it appears that there is actually an increase in the amount of paper used. This is because of the need for print outs of the information held on computer. There are a variety of different printers available. The print out they produce is known as *hard copy*.

Printers are mechanical devices and as such work more slowly than the computer. Some computers have software that directs the communication between computer and printer: this is known as a spooler. Many computers do not have this facility and you may find that you have to wait until the printer has finished before you can carry on working. Some printers have got around this problem by having their own memory. The information is sent to the printer and held there in its memory.

Printers are connected to the computer by means of a cable. There are two types of cable available.

Parallel and serial connections

Parallel cables are the most common. They are like an eight-lane motorway along which each bit is sent to the printer in parallel with the others in the byte. They all arrive at the printer at the same time. The cable has to have a strand for each bit of data. These cables often form a flat strip. However as each bit travels at a slightly different speed the length of the cable is strictly limited (up to 10 m). If the cable is too long, bits can arrive at different times.

Serial cables are used when the distances involved rule out the use of parallel cables. With a serial connection to a printer each bit follows the next one, as if along a single-lane carriageway. This means that the printer has to have information about the speed of the bits (measured in bauds) and a variety of other control details.

Impact printers

Impact printers are those that strike the page through a ribbon, like a typewriter.

Dot matrix printers Each character is made of a pattern of small dots. The more dots per character the better the quality of the print out. These printers work rapidly but are quite noisy. As the technology advances these are becoming more sophisticated and produce higher quality print outs. The advantages include the fact that they are very fast and they can handle continuous paper or separate sheets. The main disadvantages are the noise and that to produce the best quality print out does cause a marked reduction in their speed.

Line printers With this type of printer each line gets printed as one complete unit. These printers work very rapidly but are incredibly noisy and it is very difficult to work in the same room as one for any length of time.

Daisy wheel printers These printers are like their typewriter counterparts. There is a wheel (daisy wheel) with characters at the end of each spoke. The wheel rotates until the appropriate letter is in the position to strike through the ribbon. They give very good quality print out but they are very slow and noisy.

Non-impact printers

These printers produce the characters without having to strike the paper through a ribbon.

Ink jet printers These printers have a cartridge of ink which is fired at the paper. Each character is formed electrostatically. Printers of this type work very rapidly, but are quite noisy. Some ink jet printers require the use of special paper.

Laser printers Laser printers work on the principle of a photocopier. A laser beam sensitises a rotating drum where the image is formed. Powdered ink is attracted to the drum and transferred to the paper which is then heated to fix the ink. This produces very good quality print out quickly. Laser printers are very versatile as they are capable of printing text and graphics. The prices are dropping, but they are more expensive than other types of printer.

Plotters

Plotters use pens to form characters and graphics. The pens are placed in holders. Some machines allow the pen arms to move over the paper; in others the paper shunts backwards and forwards under the pen. They are used in specialised applications, for instance computer-aided design and manufacture.

Robots

Another output device is a robot. Robots are used in some factories, as part of the manufacturing process. They move forward, backward, turn so many revolutions and so on as a result of instructions given to the robot by the computer.

Speech

Speech is used as a form of output. For instance, when you phone Directory Enquiries the output from the computer comes to you as a simulated voice giving you the number you have asked for.

Magnetic tape

As with disks, tape can also be a form of output. The computer can output the results of a series of instructions to tape, so that they can be accessed at a later date.

Disks

Disks can be used as a form of output. Sometimes you will give the computer a set of instructions to perform. You may then have to go and do something else. You can get the computer to write the output from the instructions to disk. This means that you will be able to look at it later, at your convenience.

Backing store devices

The backing store talked about above comprised hard and floppy disks. There are a variety of less common devices available.

Magnetic tape and tape streamers

Information can be stored on tape and accessed later. Tapes are a cheap way of storing large amounts of information and they are commonly used with mainframe computers. As discussed above, their use is limited as they are linear storage devices and it can be difficult to find the area of interest if only a small amount of data is required from storage (p. 18).

Tape streamers are hardware devices that allow you to back up the contents of your hard disk onto a small computer tape. These tapes are generally cassettes, roughly the size of video or audio tapes. It is a fairly rapid way of being able to back up all the contents of your disk.

CD-ROM

This stands for *Compact Disk Read Only Memory*. This harnesses the technology made available from the music industry. Vast amounts of data can be stored on a compact disk. The information can be accessed and read, but it cannot be changed in any way. Encylopaedias, library catalogues and other huge databases are becoming available on CD-ROM. The drawback is that you will require a CD player to be plugged into the computer and special software to make it work.

Communications hardware

Computers can communicate with one another in a variety of different ways. Some aspects of this are discussed further in Chapter 9.

Modem

A *modem* is a device that allows two computers to communicate and share data using telephone lines. The word is an abbreviation of *mod*ulator *dem*odulator.

Telephone lines deal with analogue signals whereas computers use digital signals. The modem translates the outgoing digital signal to an analogue form so that it can be carried on the telephone line. It reverses the process at the other end.

Summary

This chapter has given you a brief description of the personal computer (PC) and the parts, or hardware, that you will come across using an 'average PC'. This description has been divided into the basic parts of the computer, as shown in Figure 1.1. There has also been some description of other hardware devices that you may come across when using computers in a variety of different situations.

The following chapter will give a brief outline of the development of the PC and subsequent chapters in this section will discuss operating systems and the different types of software that are available. This will be followed by a chapter looking at sharing data and resources.

The development of the PC | 2

Outline

Computer systems are essentially about gathering, sorting and analysing data and then outputting it in a usable format. Up to the mid 1970s the only type of computers available were mainframes or minicomputers. These were only used in the workplace by a relatively small number of individuals. They were slow and inflexible, and usually designed to cope with massive number-crunching activities such as maintaining stock lists or managing payrolls. The very idea of a personal computer in the home seemed a remote and futurist notion.

Towards the end of the decade, the revolution in silicon chip production methods meant that it became possible to mass produce small 'microcomputers', designed for single users. The arrival of cheap silicon chips unleashed an explosion of microcomputers that individuals could use to aid them in day-to-day tasks both in their workplaces and in their homes. Free to use their own personal computers to manipulate textual, numerical or graphical information, computer users were no longer tied to other people's schedules to produce a report or analyse statistics.

This chapter will discuss the genesis of the microcomputer. The discussion will commence with a brief history of mainframes and minicomputers. It will then give more detail of the development of personal computing, with particular emphasis on the IBM-compatible personal microcomputer – commonly known as the PC. The final section of the chapter will try to outline the kind of developments in personal computer technology than can be expected in the immediate future.

The development of mainframe and minicomputers

The idea of a device that would facilitate the computation of numerical information has excited the imagination of scientists and philosophers over the past two centuries, but it was only at the start of this century that it became possible to build the first working mechanically operated calculating machines. Once it became apparent that mechanically driven computing machines would always remain crude and unreliable, the attention of scientists and developers turned to the idea of developing electrically operated computing devices. It is these electronically operated devices that led directly to the computers in use today.

First generation computers

The first electrically operated computers became available in the 1940s. By today's standards they were extremely expensive and primitive. They were valve driven devices and because of this they used vast amounts of electricity. The valves in these computers often overheated or blew, so that large numbers of people were required to monitor their status and change them as required. These first generation computers were programmed using a binary coding system, known as machine language. Binary systems consist of just 1s and 0s, so programming the first generation computers was extremely tedious and difficult.

Second generation computers

The second generation computers were developed with the introduction of transistors in the 1950s and 1960s. These computers were more reliable than the earlier valve driven machines. The programs for the second generation computers were written using assembly language, a series of mnemonics which represented binary code.

Assembly language mnemonics are generally three letter abbreviations, so for instance *add* might mean addition and *mul* might mean multiply and so on. Today assembly language is used to write programs that are expected to be executed (or run) very fast, because the number of steps needed to translate from assembly language into binary is very small and therefore the computer can process them very rapidly. It is not easy to write programs in assembly language; the programmer has to give the computer very precise instructions, taking into account the internal architecture (or structure) of the computer. There are different assembly languages for the different types of microprocessors.

Third generation computers

Third generation computers were introduced with the discovery of integrated circuit technology. An integrated circuit consists of very large numbers of transistors linked together in one circuit. Third generation computers were programmed using high level languages such as FORTRAN, PASCAL and COBOL. These high level languages allow programmes to be written in a more conventional mathematical or English-like notation using a set of reserved words. Underlying these reserved words are a series of assembly language instructions so that the programmer using a high level language does not have to be so explicit about the instructions given to the computer.

Fourth and fifth generation computers

The development of further technological advances over the past two decades has led to the emergence of the fourth generation of computers. These are characterised by the so-called fourth generation languages (or 4GLs). Fourth generation languages are even more similar to natural language, and thus enable programmers to develop software very rapidly, and non-programmers to develop their own software more easily.

Fifth generation computers are the computers of the future. It is probable that these computers may make more use of expert systems, voice recognition and natural language processing (being able to process English-like statements instead of relying on more stylised computer languages).

Mainframe, mini- and microcomputers

As well as being described in terms of their evolution over time, computers traditionally have also been divided into different types depending on their size and power. Using this classification system, computers can be separated into mainframe, mini- or microcomputer categories. Initially it was very easy to make these distinctions between the different categories based on the physical size, the amount of memory, the processing power and number of users that the computer supported. Lately, however, the divisions between the classes have become somewhat more blurred.

When the first generations of mainframe computers were being developed in the 1950s they took up whole buildings or whole floors of buildings. Nowadays the same processing power can be achieved by a personal microcomputer sitting on a desk. At present mainframe computers are about the size of a couple of filing cabinets, but in spite of their smaller size, they are powerful enough to support many users at a time so they are often used to process information for an entire hospital or an educational establishment.

Minicomputers tend to be the size of photocopiers and they are designed to support several users at one time. Laboratory computer systems are often based on minicomputers.

Desktop computers or portable computers are microcomputers, and the rest of this chapter is devoted to a discussion of their history and development.

Batch and interactive mode

When using computers, another classification system to be aware of is the difference between *batch* and *interactive* mode. In batch mode the programming instructions for a particular task are submitted to the computer as a batch job. This means that once the program has started the person who submitted the job has no control over what is going on. The computer only returns control to the user once it has completed the task. If there is a mistake in the program or an error occurs while the job is running the whole job will be aborted with an appropriate error message. In hospitals with mainframe computers, a batch job is often used to update the data on the computer overnight using the information collected during the day.

By contrast, in interactive mode, the user communicates with the computer one instruction at a time. Interactive mode is a two-way process, similar to a conversation. Unlike a batch job it depends upon the user being there to prompt the computer at each appropriate step. Interactive mode is the commonest mode of communicating with microcomputers.

Many computers and computer application programs will work in either mode. For example, some GP computer systems use batch mode to search and analyse the data in the computer while still allowing a number of users to perform other interactive tasks on the computer at the same time. Some statistical application packages, used to analyse data, can be run in either batch or interactive mode.

The origins of personal computers

It has been said that if cars had miniaturised and their prices dropped at the same rate as computer technology has advanced, a Rolls-Royce would cost about £20 and fit inside a matchbox. Once microchip technology made it possible to mass produce silicon chips, it also became possible to produce microcomputers cheaply enough for the ordinary individual to buy. To meet the demand for personal computers, a number of different computer companies began designing and building personal computers. Many of the computer companies sprang up overnight, started by computer and electronics enthusiasts, some of whom were still in their teens.

With the ability to produce cheaper computer hardware came a corresponding explosion in the development of computer software for the personal computers, such as operating systems, languages, utilities and games. Soon application programs followed, allowing the personal computer user to manipulate different types of information – word processors for textual information, spreadsheets for numerical information and so on.

In the initial stages of the personal computer revolution, each of the companies who began building personal computers and designing software did so using their own proprietary design, because the technology itself was so new there were no standard systems to rely on. With the plethora of different and mainly incompatible products available, the situation for the consumer became rather confusing. Which type of personal computer and software should he or she choose? There were Apples, BBCs and Sinclair Spectrum computers as well as many others, all utilising varying types of software and hardware.

Eventually the giant computer company IBM, which up to that point had been standing on the sidelines, decided it too would produce a personal computer. As time was short, they concentrated on buying-in electronic components that had already been developed, or were being developed. The main 'bought-in' components of this IBM personal computer (or the PC as it came to be known), were the CPU and the operating system.

The development of the IBM PC

At the time it brought out its personal computer, IBM was by far the biggest computer company in the world. Indeed because of its pre-eminence, there was a saying that 'No one ever got fired for buying IBM'. IBM's personal computer soon became the popular choice, and because it was built from standard non-proprietary components, other computer companies soon began producing very similar machines. These personal computers became known as *IBM-compatible PCs* or *IBM clones*.

At the start of the PC explosion triggered by the arrival of the IBM PC and its clones, it is fair to say that nobody predicted the extent of the computer revolution that would ensue. Because of this lack of foresight, the first PCs were produced without certain limitations in the original technology being resolved. Unfortunately, however, to understand fully why these limitations created such problems (which are only now being resolved), it is necessary to understand a little more of what goes on inside an IBM-compatible PC.

There are several essential components to any computer, as discussed in Chapter 1. The first of these components is the central processing unit or CPU. This contains the chip which perform the calculations on which the whole functioning of the computer is based, and the computer memory which stores information that the chip requires on a second-to-second basis as it operates. These basic hardware components (and other hardware devices) are controlled by software known as the computer's *operating system*. Chapter 1 has already discussed PC computer hardware, and Chapter 3 will discuss PC operating systems in more detail. This chapter will concentrate on discussing the interaction between these two components.

The 8086/8088 chip, PC-DOS and the one megabyte limit

When IBM introduced its first PC over 10 years ago it had to find a chip and a new operating system for it. The chips were bought in from a company called Intel, and the first IBM PCs were known as XT personal computers (the XT stood for eXtra Technology) because they used the newer 8088 chips developed by Intel. These 8086 chips had a 16 bit capacity and so were more powerful than the original first generation chip, an 8 bit chip known as the 8088. Although the 8088 chip was regarded as a fairly powerful chip at that time, the internal design of these chips meant that they could not access more than 2^{20} bytes of memory (or one megabyte) because there were only 20 channels linking the 8088 chip to the memory (2^{20} bytes equals 1 048 576 bytes or one megabyte).

At the time that IBM released its first PCs, it chose a small company, Microsoft, to produce the operating system. In turn Microsoft bought in an operating system based on a design created by someone else, made some alterations, and named it the PC Disk Operating System or PC-DOS. Later on, as Microsoft grew into a large company in its own right and sold the operating system to all the other PC clone manufacturers, this operating system became more commonly known as MS-DOS. (Nowadays these operating systems are collectively known as DOS).

This DOS operating system for the first generation of IBM PCs was also designed with the same internal limitation as the first generation of chips – it could only 'see' one megabyte of memory. At that time, most computer experts did not think that this design limitation would be a problem, as there were already many other types of microcomputers running quite well with 128 kilobytes of memory – or only an eighth of a megabyte. At that time the cost of all hardware components including the memory chips themselves was still fairly high. This first megabyte of memory in a PC, which can be addressed by both DOS and the 8086/8088 chips, is known as *conventional* or *base memory*.

Using memory

As the original allocation of a whole megabyte of memory seemed so generous to the designers of DOS, they imposed another limitation. They split the mega-byte into two sections, a lower section of 640 kilobytes and an upper section of 384 kilobytes and reserved the upper portion for the computer's own use. This only left 640 kilobytes of lower memory for application programs to use.

Lower memory. Because of the design of the original chip in the first IBM PC, and the first version of DOS, the 640 kilobyte lower portion of conventional or base memory remains the most accessible portion of computer memory. Many DOS application programs can only run in lower conventional or base memory. However, this space is not entirely free even before any application programs are loaded, because certain essential functions must always be present in RAM at all times for the computer itself to function. These functions include a portion of the operating system itself, and the little programs that control how the computer interacts with its peripheral devices (such as the keyboard, mouse and VDU)

Upper memory. The upper 384 kilobyte section of base memory is reserved for the computer's own use. For example, 128 kilobytes are needed for the Read Only Memory (ROM) BIOS, and 128 kilobytes are reserved for output to the visual display unit (VDU). Other sections in upper memory were reserved by the first version of DOS for future use by the computer. Upper memory can be divided into contiguous 'chunks' called *upper memory blocks* or UMBs.

Using memory for essential functions

When a PC is switched on it boots up, i.e. essential DOS files are loaded from the hard disk into the lower portion of the memory so that they are always accessible while the computer is on. If these files are not present on the hard disk, they must be present on a floppy disk that is sitting in the A: drive as the computer is switched on. A floppy that carries these files is therefore known as a bootable floppy disk or a system disk.

The files that are loaded into the memory include COMMAND.COM, the file that contains the essential DOS functions discussed above. This is discussed further in Chapter 3. Small programs, called device drivers, that contain instructions to allow the computer to control the various hardware devices such as the keyboard, mouse and VDU, are also loaded into the memory. Other files that may remain in the memory are TSRs (Terminate and Stay Resident). These are programs that remain in memory and are always available to the user, from any application program. They are discussed in more detail in Chapter 4.

Using memory for computer programs

The main function of RAM is to make it possible to run the actual application programs which are the primary reason for using a computer in the first place. In general, it is not possible or desirable to get an entire application programme into RAM, so most application programs are designed in a modular fashion so that only a certain number of files from the application program are held in RAM at one time: other files are called into RAM as required.

In essence, the amount of free RAM and the power of the chip determine the size of application programs that can be run, the number of application programs that can be run simultaneously and the speed that the application programs can be run at. Although the first chips, the first versions of DOS and the first PCs were designed to work with a single megabyte of RAM, it is self-evident that running application programs faster, or running more sophisticated application programs is always desirable. Chapter 9 will discuss the desirability of being able to open more than one application program at a time. The rest of this chapter will cover the hardware and software developments that have been able to improve the speed and power of PC chips, and increase the amount of RAM available to them

Techniques to free up conventional memory

As the designers of application software strained against the 640k limit of lower conventional or base memory, other designers of computer hardware and software raced ahead to try to find ways of maximising the amount of free memory in this area.

Expanded memory. This solution to increasing the amount of memory under the one megabyte limit was developed in the mid-to late 1980s, most notably by a group of software companies incorporating Lotus, Intel and Microsoft (LIM). The method employed to create extra memory used a process known as bank switching or *paging*. This process of paging requires three components. First a 64 kilobyte chunk is identified in the area above the conventional memory which is then divided into four 16 kilobyte regions called *page frames*. Secondly, either an additional expanded memory card (*Expanded Memory System* or EMS) or extra memory chips are installed in the computer, and thirdly a piece of memory manager software that allows mapping of 16 kilobyte pages of memory from the EMS card into the page frame. When running a program that supports expanded memory the data is loaded into the memory of the EMS. When the PC needs to access the data contained within the expanded memory it is rerouted by the EMM through the page frame to the data.

Application programs use this expanded memory for storing data while the programs are running. The system has to be told that the memory management software exists. This is done by adding a line, or instructions, into the CONFIG.SYS file (Chapter 3).

Extended memory is the large storage area that lies above the one megabyte limit. Programs that use extended memory are loaded into conventional memory and the program loads its data into the extended memory. When the program needs to access the data stored in the extended memory it does so more directly without having to do any of the page swapping done by expanded memory. For this reason it is much faster.

To access the extended memory there is a special software device driver, known as an extended memory manager. As with expanded memory the system has to be told that the memory manager software exists. This is also done by adding a line or instruction into the CONFIG.SYS file (Chapter 3).

The 80286 chip and extended memory

In 1982 the 286 chip was introduced. PCs based on the 286 chip and above became known as PC AT (the AT stands for Advanced Technology). The 286 chip was faster and more powerful than the 8086/8088 chip used in the first PCs. In addition, it could also 'see' more than one megabyte of memory. This ability to address the additional memory was accomplished by linking the 286 chip to the memory by 24 channels instead of the previous 20. Therefore the 286 chip could access 2^{24} bytes of memory (or approximately 16 megabytes). Unlike earlier chips, the 286 chip can run in two modes, *real mode* and *protected mode*.

Real mode

In real mode the 286 chip acts just like a fast 8086/8088 chip, but it has two limitations. It can still only address one megabyte of memory, and it can really only run one program at a time. This mode of operation was retained by the chip's designers so that programs originally written for the 8086/8088 chip could still run on the 286.

Protected mode

In protected mode the 286 chip can address up to 16 megabytes of memory. The memory lying above the one megabyte limit is known as extended memory to distinguish it from the expanded memory discussed earlier. However, in this situation the limitation of DOS come into play, as DOS itself cannot access memory above the one megabyte limit.

Using extended memory

Most modern application programs can benefit from additional memory. More memory means that the program can run faster, and perform more ambitious tasks. As expanded memory predated extended memory, it can be helpful to configure extended memory as expanded memory, especially when using application programs that are designed to use expanded memory.

Using extended memory for RAM disks

Another use for extended memory is as a 'virtual' disk drive or RAM disk. Virtual in computing terminology is used to describe something that can simulate the functions of something else. A virtual disk drive is an area created in memory to act as a small disk drive which programs can use to store temporary information while they are working. The advantage of a RAM disk is that it can speed up some programs' operations. The disadvantages are that a RAM disk can reduce the memory available for programmes and, as discussed in Chapter 1, information held in RAM is lost if the computer experiences a sudden loss of power.

The 386 chip

The first 32 bit chip was the 386 chip, but fairly soon after its introduction a cut down version, the 386sx, was released. The 386 chip uses 32 channels to communicate with other parts of the computer. Like the full 386 chip (or 386dx as it is sometimes known), the 386sx can process 32 bits of information internally, but it communicates with the other computer peripherals via a 16 bit data communication channel. 386sx chips are used in computers with a lower specification and are now considered the entry level chips for anyone purchasing new computer equipment.

The 486 Chip

The 486 chip is the most recent chip to be introduced. Like the 386 chip, the 486 chip is also a 32 bit chip but it is even more fast and powerful. It also has a cut down version, the 486sx. With the advent of the 486 chip the situation has grown more confused: there are now a number of ways of speeding up a PC by adding additional chips to the motherboard – chips to double the speed of existing 486 chips, chips to convert 486sx chips to full 486 chips and so on. In fact, because of the rapid pace of technology, hardware manufactures are now producing upgradable PCs – PCs where many of the components can be replaced as new versions of hardware are released.

The 586 or Pentium Chip

This chip has recently been introduced by Intel. For copyright reasons it is known as the Pentium. All indications suggest that it will remain relatively expensive in the immediate future so it is unlikely to become the standard chip for most PCs for a while.

32 bit chips and multi-tasking operating systems

DOS was originally developed in a great hurry because of the tight schedule that IBM insisted on for producing the first IBM PC. In fact, the version of DOS was named 86-QDOS by its inventor, QDOS standing for the Quick and Dirty operating System. DOS was not meant to have the pre-eminent role that it has today – if it had been, its internal limitations would never have been allowed to get past the first post.

At the time that DOS for IBM PC was being developed by Microsoft, another computer company (Apple) was developing its own personal computer. It used a different chip (made by Motorola), and in contrast to the IBM PC, the Apple personal computer began life with a *graphical user interface* (GUI), and a *multi-tasking operating system* that had no problems addressing more than one megabyte of memory. In spite of this advantage, other commercial considerations meant that this superior type of personal computer design did not gain the foothold that the IBM PC and DOS did.

As early as the mid-1980s both IBM and Microsoft began to think about producing a better operating system to run on PCs that would incorporate the GUI/multi-tasking advantages of the Apple operating system. The term 'graphical' when applied to computer software (as in graphical user interface or GUI) implies that the software has a menu and picture-based interface rather than a text-based interface. The use of a GUI will be discussed in more detail in Chapter 4. The ability to multi-task will be discussed in Chapter 9.

Multi-tasking with the PC

In pursuit of a multi-tasking operating system, IBM initially produced an operating system called Topview, which never became widely accepted. Then, in conjunction with Microsoft, it moved on to developing a multi-tasking operating system with a graphical user interface known as OS/2. Microsoft also continued to work on its own separate multi-tasking/graphical user interface enhancement to DOS which it called Windows. The first version of Windows was not a success, but later versions have become very popular. OS/2 has also been developed as a GUI/multi-tasking operating system. These are discussed in more detail in Chapters 4 and 9.

The future

It is notoriously difficult to predict the future in the fast-changing world of computer technology. Indeed, when the mighty Goliath of IBM first approached the puny David of Microsoft to buy an operating system, it is probable that no one could have predicted the role reversal in profits and influence that would occur within the space of less than 15 years. In the mid-1970s when IBM and Microsoft were collaborating on their first personal computers, these computers were using 8 bit chips, able to process 8 bits of information at any one time. The first computer also had no disk drives and less than one megabyte of memory. Programs were small enough to be housed on the low capacity floppy disks along with the operating system.

It is evident to even most computer-phobic eye that has been a lot of change since these early days. Indeed the pace of change in information technology in general has been so great that we are probably living through the electronic equivalent of the industrial revolution. The arrival of every new chip, the unveiling of each enhancement to the operating systems, the release of new versions of software, has made the previously introduced new technology seem old hat within a very short space of time. Therefore, even at the risk of appearing foolish in the very near future, the next section will attempt to outline the changes just ahead on the horizon.

Future chip developments

Up to now all the IBM-based PCs have used chips based on the original 8086/8088 chip, and the majority of these chips have been made by one company, Intel, or made by other companies working under licence. However, making chips for the mass market is obviously a very profitable enterprise. Other companies have therefore tried to move into this market by trying to design equivalent chips, by a process known as 'reverse engineering'

At present there are a number of different Intel and Intel-like chips on the market for PCs. They are the so-called CISC chips, or complex instruction set chips. The latest of these is the Pentium. The next generation of operating systems to run on the PC could make use of so-called RISC chips (reduce instruction set chips). RISC chips are currently used to run multi-tasking operating systems like Unix on mainframes and minicomputers. In many situations they are much more powerful than CISC chips, so powerful in fact that it has been inefficient to use them in PCs because of other limitations inherent in PC hardware and software. However, with the advances in PC operating systems it well may be possible to use RISC chips in a PC.

The Alpha Chip

Intel-like chips have dominated the PC market but the Alpha chip represents a new departure. Unlike the Intel chips it is a 64 bit super fast microprocessor. The manufacturer, DEC, has developed the chip at great expense and it is unlikely to be superseded within the next ten years because of its inherent ability to be enhanced. The Alpha chip can run a number of different operating systems making it more versatile than the Intel chips.

Future operating system developments

As the operating systems develop there is more emphasis placed on allowing PC users to perform more than one task at a time. There is also a move to produce systems that will allow computers to link together. This is discussed in more detail in Chapter 9.

The requirement for an operating system is not peculiar to micro- or personal computers — mainframes and minicomputers also require an operating system. However, unlike those discussed so far, the operating systems for most mainframes and minicomputers are proprietary — in other words they are specific to each make of mainframe and minicomputer. The disadvantage of proprietary operating systems for the consumer is that buying a computer with such an operating system often locks the purchaser into a particular supplier's hardware and software products. For this reason computer suppliers are finding it harder and harder to sell computer hardware that requires a proprietary operating system.

There is an operating system for the mainframe and minicomputer which is non-proprietary, probable because it was originally developed in a university rather than a commercial setting. This operating system is known as *Unix* Because Unix was developed to run on a number of different types of computers, and because of the rapid advances of PC hardware technology, it is now possible to run Unix as a multi-user operating system on a PC. As Unix is an older operating system, there is also a great deal of experience of using it on mainframes and minicomputers. These factors, coupled with the fact that it is regarded as an 'open', or non-proprietary operating system, mean Unix now appears to be the one of the main contenders in the battle for a standard multi-user operating system for all types of computers.

Unix is inherently an open system, but at present there are still a number of different proprietary versions of it on the market, which remain incompatible with each other to a greater or lesser extent. For the non-expert user intending to run only a single PC or a small multi-user system, Unix, although powerful, is also an extremely difficult operating system to use and, in comparison to the wealth of software available for DOS, Windows or even OS/2, the software available for Unix is sparse, difficult to use and relatively expensive.

Windows NT

DOS is a 16 bit operating system; Windows NT, which has been developed by Microsoft, is a 32 bit operating system. Unlike Windows, which requires DOS as the operating system, Windows NT is an operating system in its own right. It can run DOS and Windows programs as well as running software designed for Unix. As well as running on Intel chips it can make use of the new Alpha chip and other chips, not discussed in this book, which currently run Unix. Windows NT has improved data security which makes it more acceptable to large organisations. This together with its other strengths makes it likely to become a direct competitor to Unix in the multi-user market.

Summary

This chapter has outlined the development of the PC. The predominance of IBM PCs and DOS over other better hardware design and rival operating systems indicates that evolution rather than revolution is probable the way ahead. The future solutions will be those that do not force users to cope with massive changes in either the hardware or software that they are used to. For these reasons the future is likely to feature the DOS-based IBM PC.

Like all large organisations were the acquisition, analysis and dissemination of information is becoming increasingly important, the Health Service will be profoundly affected by these developments in computer technology. The immediate future for the Health Service will probably lie in the retention of mainframes and minicomputers as information repositories, but with the addition of a shell of PCs, allowing users easy access to the manipulation of the data that they require on a daily basis

The following chapter looks at DOS in more detail and subsequent chapters will look at the different types of application packages that are available for DOS-based machines. The final chapter in this section looks at sharing data and linking computers together.

3 | Introduction to the Disk Operating System (DOS)

The previous chapter introduced the concept of an operating system. This chapter will provide an introduction to operating systems, specifically the Disk Operating System (DOS), although others will be mentioned. DOS is the most common operating system found on IBM-compatible personal computers in business and in the Health Service. For this reason it is dealt with in detail here. Many of the commands available within application packages (software) that you may have access to are based upon DOS commands. An understanding of the basic principles will enhance your use of application packages.

What is an operating system?

An operating system is a group of programs that allow you to use the computer. The operating system performs such tasks as creating files, running programs and printing documents. It is a housekeeper for the computer. It manages files and data throughout the system and serves as an interface between you, the program and the rest of your computer. Almost anything you do with a computer will be done through the operating system. Figure 3.1 shows this schematically. The computer and its associated software can be thought of as a series of skins or shells. At the heart is the hardware; surrounding this is the first shell which is the operating system. Application packages then form the next layer of shells. In some cases the first layer may be a user-friendly application package, such as Windows (Chapter 4). The further layers will be the application packages such as a database, spreadsheet or word processor. All of these are discussed in subsequent chapters.

The operating system as translator

You can think of the operating system as a translator. The computer understands binary (1s and Os), you speak English. Without a translator there is no way the

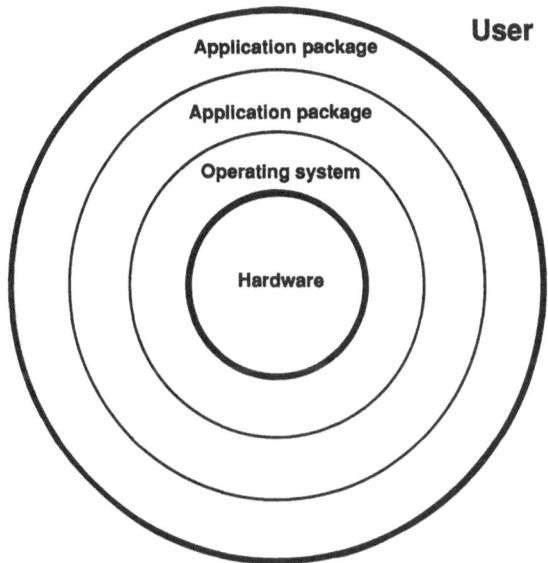

Figure 3.1 How the operating system interacts with hardware, other types of software and the user. There can be any number of application package shells. At times when the user is directly using the operating system there will be no outer shells.

two can communicate. The operating system acting as a translator translates the English-like statements which you type into binary. The computer can then execute the instructions given. The operating system will then translate the binary output from the computer into English so that you can see and understand the results of the action which you have asked for.

Different operating systems

There are a variety of different operating systems which you may come across, for example, Pick, VME and VM/IS. OS/2, Unix and Windows NT have already been mentioned in Chapter 2 and there are others. They perform the same tasks as DOS, but the commands involved will be different. Some operating systems allow several people to use the computer at the same time (multi-user) or allow users to perform more than one task at the same time (multi-tasking). This is discussed more fully in Chapter 9.

Disk Operating System – DOS

There are various different types of DOS. MS-DOS stands for Microsoft DOS, the version of DOS which is released by the Microsoft company. PC-DOS is Personal Computer DOS issued by IBM. DR-DOS is Digital Research DOS issued by the company Digital Research. AM-DOS is Amstrad DOS issued by Amstrad and so on. If you understand the principles of MS-DOS and someone asks if you can use PC-DOS the answer is yes as they are broadly the same, with corresponding functions.

After the name MS-DOS or PC-DOS there will be a number like 3.1, 3.3, 4.0, 5.0 or 6.0. These numbers refer to the version of DOS with which you are working. As problems become evident with DOS or refinements are added, new versions are issued. This is reflected in the version number. Anything you can do in versions 3.1 DOS can be done in version 5.0. However, there are some things in version 5.0 which are not available in version 3.1. Generally when you buy some software to run on the computer it will tell you that it expects the facilities of a particular version of DOS. What this means is that you can run the software on a computer with that or higher versions of DOS, but not with any lower version. The advantages of higher versions have been discussed in Chapter 2.

What DOS does

When the computer is turned on the system boots up. That means the computer is started up and gets ready for you to use it. Part of the booting up instructions are held in the Read Only Memory or ROM of the computer. Part of these instructions will say to the computer, if there is a floppy disk in disk drive A: have a look and get more instructions from there. During the start up procedure the computer will look at the floppy disk drive; if there is more than one floppy disk drive it will only look at the one labelled A:, which is generally the disk drive at the top or on the right hand side. If there is no disk in A: the Read Only Memory instructions tell the machine to find the remainder of the starting up instructions which are stored on the hard disk. These instructions include loading up some of the operating system commands into memory. Some of the DOS commands are stored in a special file called COMMAND.COM, which is loaded into memory. These commands are known as *internal* commands and they will remain in the memory of the computer the whole time it is switched on. Other DOS commands, that do not remain in the memory the whole time but are retrieved from the disk as necessary, are known as *external* commands.

If the computer does not have a hard disk you must put a special *system disk* into the floppy disk drive when you switch on. If there is no disk in the floppy disk drive or the disk is one that does not contain the specific start up instructions you will get an error message on the screen saying: 'insert system disk into drive and press any key to continue'. If you do not do this you will get no further and you will be unable to use the machine. There must be an operating system in the memory of the machine for you to be able to use the computer. As the operating system loads into the memory, various messages will probably be displayed on the screen until finally a prompt will be displayed.

Entering DOS commands and case sensitivity

DOS is what is termed *'case insensitive'*. This means that you can type in upper or lower case letters or a mixture of the two. The machine will interpret the commands in the same way. Most software packages are *case sensitive*. This means that they will interpret something typed in upper case differently from the same item typed in lower case.

In what follows in this chapter the commands that you will have to type have been printed bold and in upper case, just to distinguish them from the remainder of the text. You must type them exactly as they appear. Any keys that you have to press, for instance <ENTER>, are enclosed in <> brackets.

Prompt

The prompt displayed on the screen usually gives the letter of the drive from which DOS was booted up. This is known as the *default drive*. If you have put the starting up instructions on a floppy in disk drive A: the prompt will contain the letter A. If the instructions have come from the hard disk the letter C will appear in the prompt.

The prompt consists of the letter followed by a colon, a backslash and a greater than sign (e.g.C:\>). After the greater than sign is a flashing line which is known as the cursor. The letter is part of the disk drive name. So that the machine can distinguish between a letter you might type from the keyboard and the disk drive name, there is a colon which is also part of the drive name. The backslash is explained below. The greater than sign indicates that this is the end of the prompt. The flashing line, the cursor, indicates where anything you type at the keyboard will be displayed on the screen. Sometimes you may see this kind of entry, typing at the prompt, referred to as *command line entry*.

Disk drives

By convention DOS labels disk drives as letters. A: and B: are reserved for floppy disk drives. If you have one then you only have A:. if you have two then you have A: and B:. C: is reserved for the hard disk. Sometimes the hard disk is also labelled D:. This is because some versions of DOS are unable to support a hard disk larger than a maximum size of 32 megabytes. If you have a hard disk which is 40 megabytes, although it is all the one hard disk, it is logically divided into C: and D:. C: has 32 megabytes and D: has 8 megabytes. In the later versions of DOS, from DOS 4.0 onwards, the operating system can handle a hard disk which is larger than 32 megabytes and therefore the need for a D: drive has been eliminated.

If your machine has another disk drive attached to it, this is often labelled E: for external disk drive. So for instance if you wanted to add a $5\frac{1}{4}$" disk drive to a machine which had a $3\frac{1}{2}$" disk drive then that $5\frac{1}{4}$" disk drive may be labelled E: to signify the external drive. If your computer is linked into a network you are able to access the hard disk of the central machine or file server. This is discussed again in Chapter 9. Not all of these will be available in any one machine, but there are a variety of different disk drives available.

Changing disk drive

If you wish to change disk drives you simply type in the name of the drive that you want to look at. For instance, if you wanted to have a look at the contents of a floppy disk you would tell the machine to change disk drives by typing A: followed by ENTER. If you do not press the ENTER key the machine does not know that you have finished giving the command and it will do nothing. After you have pressed the ENTER key you will notice that the light comes on at the disk drive. This indicates that the machine is now looking at the disk in the disk drive. The prompt on the screen will change to A:\> (or B:\>) depending on which drive you have asked the machine to look at.

Electronic filing

Directories

If you want the machine to look at the contents of the disk you have to issue an appropriate DOS command. To tell the machine to give you a list of what is on the disk the command is DIR: this is short for directory. What you are actually saying to the machine is list the contents of this disk, on the screen. You will get a list of things contained on the disk. In this chapter we are going to be working to an example which is shown in Figure 3.2, the directory tree. The structure is actually an upside down tree and in this respect is like a family tree. The top of the tree is known as the root and that is symbolised by the backslash (\). In the prompt we looked at earlier, therefore, the backslash following say A: indicates that the machine is looking at the floppy disk drive A: and is at the root, which is the top of this tree structure.

In Figure 3.2 are various boxes which are called *directories*. The boxes have contents which are called *files*. With a paper system, if you practise a chaotic method of filing you will probably have to search through many piles of papers on your desk or in your filing cabinets before you can find anything. This obviously wastes a lot of your time. If, however, you file all your correspondence in a logical order it will be more a straightforward and quicker task to find anything. The same holds true of electronic filing.

A 40 megabyte hard disk actually has space for thousands of files to be stored upon it. If there is no organised system for storing these files retrieving them at a later date can be very difficult. This is especially true if you have forgotten what you called the file. To overcome this the operating system forces you to be fairly

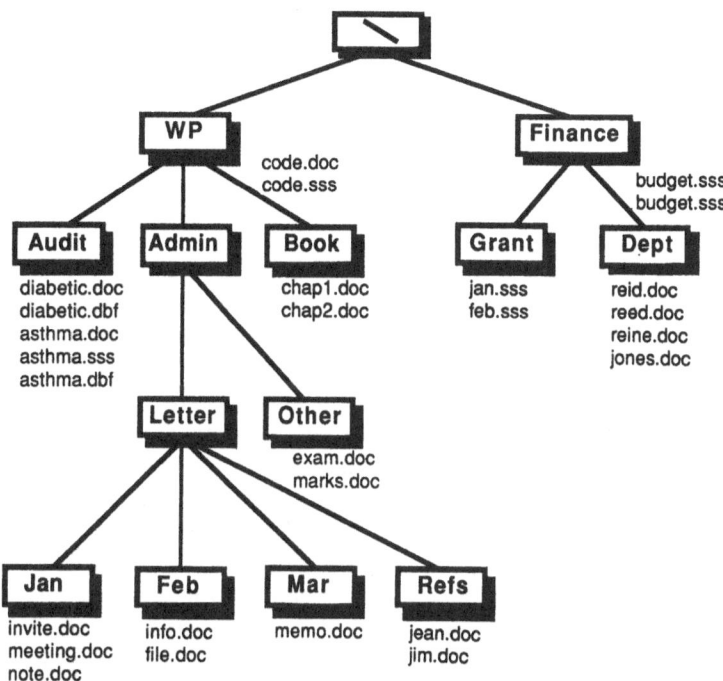

Figure 3.2 The directory tree. This is the arrangement of directories and files that will be used throughout this chapter. Each individual can make directory trees to suit their own ways of working.

organised about the way you store the information on the disk. The disk can actually be likened to a filing system in a filing cabinet. Inside each drawer in a filing cabinet there are a series of pouches into which you place documents which are related. If you think of the disk as the drawer of the filing cabinet, each of the boxes or directories can be seen as a pouch inside the drawer into which you place related items. The analogy really stops there because on a disk you can have subdirectories within directories to as many levels as you like. Obviously you would not put pouches inside pouches in a filing cabinet drawer. However the basic principle is the same. A directory is really a box or a pouch into which related documents, or files, are placed.

In the directory tree structure shown in Figure 3.2 there are a number of directories. Directory names are decided upon by you, the user. They can be between one and eight characters long. It is a good idea to name them appropriately and to keep them as short as possible, to minimise typing.

The finance directory has two subdirectories, GRANT and DEPT. The WP directory has three subdirectories ADMIN, AUDIT and BOOK. ADMIN and LETTER also have subdirectories. The level of complexity of the tree structure will depend on your own needs.

If asked to provide a copy of a letter sent in January, all you have to do is move from the WP directory into the ADMIN directory. From here move to the LETTER directory and then into JAN directory. You will have narrowed down the area on the disk that needs to be searched to retrieve the document. This is especially useful if you have forgotten the name you gave the file.

To see the contents of a directory (DIR)

The DOS command DIR instructs the machine to give a listing of what is on the disk. It shows the contents of the directory you happen to be in at the time, the current directory, on the screen. Each directory has its own contents page. The list on the screen is a copy of the list on this contents page. The contents page for the root directory allows a finite number of entries. This number will vary depending on your own computer set-up. If you try to save a file when the root directory is full the operating system will tell you that the disk is full up. What it actually means is that there is no more space on the contents page (also known as the *file allocation table* or FAT) for the directory. By having directories or subdirectories each of these will then have their own contents page. Only the name of the directory will appear in the contents page of its parent. All of the contents will be masked from the parent. This will free up spaces in the contents table to allow more files or directories to be stored in the current directory.

The contents page is essential for you to be able to access information from a disk. Giving the name of a file in which you are interested causes the machine to actually look in the contents page for the name of the file. Once it has found it, there is an instruction that tells the machine whereabouts on the disk the information is stored. If the name of the file is not included on the contents page the machine will be unable to retrieve it.

Files

We have seen that directories have names with between one and eight characters. If we look at the files you will see that their names are actually more complicated. They come in three parts. These names can be likened to the name of a person. There is a first name, a middle name and the surname. The first name is between one and eight characters long and you choose it when you decide what you want to call the file. You will probably find that you become very uninspired when you have to think about different file names. The second part of the file name is a full stop which is the same for all files. Unfortunately when you ask the machine to list the files it does not show the full stop. When you use the operating system and you want to look at particular files, or use various operating system commands on the files, you must put the full stop in. The final part of the name, the surname, is also called the extension. Not all files have an extension but generally there is an extension present. It has between one and three letters. The analogy to people still holds. A surname can sometimes tell you something about the person concerned. With files the surname or extension can sometimes tell you something about the contents of the file. Looking at the directory tree in the diagram you will see that there are various files present in the directories. Some of them have got the surname or extension 'DOC' which is short for document. This tells you that the file was produced in a word processor which automatically puts the extension 'DOC' on the files. In the directory named FINANCE you will see there are files with different extensions, like 'SSS' AND 'SSC'. These were created by a spreadsheet, hence 'SS.' The 'C' means that the file is a chart, or graph and the 'S' means that it is a spreadsheet. In the AUDIT directory you will see that there are a variety of different surnames. ASTHMA.DB is actually a database. ASTHMA.F is a form, to allow data to be entered into the database.

When looking at the listings of the files present in a directory then, you can tell something about them if you have a little knowledge about the meanings of the extensions.

Although you are able to choose the names of your files and directories you may run into problems when using some of the special characters. Names should not contain spaces, commas, backslashes, asterisks, question marks, plus, equals or full stops. The latter are present as the middle name of the file only. If you find that DOS will not accept other characters, check with your DOS manual.

In the root directory there are two subdirectories and some files. There are two special files – AUTOEXEC.BAT and CONFIG.SYS – which are used in the staring up or booting up process for the computer. It is of some value to understand what the contents of these two files mean.

To see the contents of a file (TYPE)

To look at the contents of a file the DOS command is TYPE. All you have to do at the prompt is key the word TYPE, leave a space and then put in the name of the file you wish to look at.

CONFIG.SYS

The CONFIG.SYS file is a special file involved in the booting up process for the computer. Its name means CONFIGure the SYStem. At the prompt (A:\>) use the DOS command to display the contents of the file on the screen.

TYPE CONFIG.SYS <ENTER>

What you will see is something like this:

    files=30
    buffers=20
    country=044

Let us take this one line at a time.

Files = command This command tells the machine that up to 30 files can be opened at one time. The operating system, and other software packages, group commands together in files. There is a file that allows the computer to talk to a printer, another that allows the keyboard to communicate with the computer and so on. All of these files have to be opened, i.e. in the computer memory, while the machine is switched on. Upon loading a piece of software the instructions that allow the machine to act as a word processor, database, spreadsheet etc, are stored in files. When you open any document to edit that is another file open. If you issue a command that is not located in a currently open file another file of instructions has to be opened. You can see that the number of files open can keep increasing. By stating in the CONFIG.SYS file that files = 30 the machine can open up to 30 files. If you issue a command that will require a thirty-first file to open, the machine must close one of the files already opened.

Stating how many files can be opened allows the machine's memory to be used to hold open files but also to be used for other purposes as well. If the total memory of the computer was occupied with open files the machine would be unable to do any other work. Thirty files seems to be a reasonable compromise that most people work with. You may find that your machine is working very slowly if it is having to swap files in and out of memory very often. By increasing the number of files open, in this command, you may be able to increase the performance of your system.

Some packages need a large number of files to be opened in the process of opening themselves. You may get an error message if they are unable to get started properly. To deal with this you may simply need to go into your CONFIG.SYS file (through the word processor or DOS editor) and change the files= command so that you increase the number of files that are open.

Buffers = command As you open files they are first stored in intermediate storage areas (or buffers) before becoming available in the memory. The more buffers present the faster the machine can perform. However, if all of the available memory is taken up with buffers the machine is unable to perform other tasks. Buffers=20 appears to be a good compromise that most people are happy with.

Country = command The next line in the display is country=044. This is the international telephone dialling code for Great Britain. This therefore tells the machine that you are in Great Britain. In Britain you will require a pound sign and the date order should show the day of the month before the month of the year. Provided you know the relevant telephone dialling code, you can tell the computer that you are in any country of your choice; unless told otherwise, the computer will assume it is in America.

Any other lines in the CONFIG.SYS file are generally instructions to the machine about the way in which the memory is configured. These are command lines which are usually entered into this file when the computer leaves the factory. They are not things that you usually have to change. If you do change the memory configuration of your machine you will probably receive instructions detailing any changes that have to be made to this file.

AUTOEXEC.BAT

The next file to look at is AUTOEXEC.BAT. This is short for AUTOmatically EXECuted BATch file. Batch use of the computer was explained in Chapter 2 (pp. 25). Sometimes it is quite useful to have batch files, that contain lists of instructions for the computer to follow. AUTOEXEC.BAT is a rather special batch file because it is automatically executed if it is present. (If it is not present it does not matter.) With other batch files, which always have the extension 'BAT' for batch, the computer has to be given a command to execute them (or perform the instructions).

Like the previous example, to look at the contents of the CONFIG.SYS file, the DOS command required is TYPE at the prompt C:\>

TYPE AUTOEXEC.BAT <ENTER>

The file displayed will look something like the following:

```
@echo off
path=C:\;C:\WP;C:\FINANCE
PROMPT $P$G
KEYB UK
echo on
```

Echo command The first line says 'echo off' and the last line says 'echo on'. *Echo* is the jargon for displaying the prompt or the current command on the screen. You will have noticed that when you type from the keyboard everything you type appears, or echoes, on the screen. Once you have got a batch file that you know works, the last thing you need is to have your screen littered up with each command as the computer executes it. Turning the echo off will stop the commands appearing on the screen. The @ before echo off means that the command itself is not shown on the screen.

Path command The next line is a path command: path=C:\;C:\WP; C:\FINANCE. This indicates to the operating system that on the hard disk there are directories present. In this case the directories are called WP and FINANCE. This allows the operating system to have a global picture of the directory tree. This can be very useful. For instance there may be a command in the FINANCE directory that you wish to use. To issue a command you generally have to be in the directory in which it resides. If you happened to be in the WP directory and wanted a command that was active in FINANCE you would have to change directory and then give the command. The path command in the AUTOEXEC.BAT file removes this need. The computer will search each directory named in the path command for any commands typed in.

Prompt command Next is the prompt command: PROMPT PG. This is the command to tell DOS to put a particular prompt on the screen. The PG is the instruction to include the path which was followed to get to the current point. If you change from the hard disk to the floppy disk drive the prompt will change from C:\> to A:\>. The machine was looking at the root directory of these particular disks, signified by the backslash immediately before the greater than sign. As you change directory and move into other directories their names appear in the prompt. If your chosen directory is several levels down, if you have to move through several subdirectories to get to it, the names of all the subdirectories would also be present in the prompt.

Changing the prompt The prompt can be anything you like. You can change the PG to any message you want. So if you wanted your computer to say 'have a nice day', you can issue the command

    PROMPT have a nice day.

This will appear on the screen where, at the moment, it says C:\>. If you change the prompt in the AUTOEXEC.BAT file it will be changed each time you turn the machine on. If you type at the current prompt your new prompt will appear until you turn the machine off. When you turn on again the prompt will be in its original form. This is because it has followed the prompt command in AUTOEXEC.BAT.

Keyboard command The next command is KEYB UK. This is instructing the machine that you will be using a UK keyboard. If you do not specify the country the machine will use the US keyboard layout. Keyboard layouts are slightly different between the different countries. The letters themselves are in the same place in English speaking nations, but some of the peripheral characters may change position. It is rather annoying for someone who can touch type to find keys behaving unexpectedly. Using a UK keyboard allows you to use the pound sign (£) if there is one on the keyboard.

That is all of the commands in the file illustrated here. However you can put in any command you like. For instance you may need to give certain instructions to a printer, each time you switch on your computer, before you can use it. It is best to automate this process by placing the instructions in the AUTOEXEC.BAT file. They will be done automatically every time you turn the machine on. Once you have sorted out the file so that it works, you never have to worry about these instructions again.

Any changes that you make to the AUTOEXEC.BAT file, while using the computer, will not come into effect until you reboot the machine. As the computer starts up it will read the AUTOEXEC.BAT file and execute the new commands.

Other batch files

Your computer may have a series of other batch files which are available to you. One of the most common uses of batch files is to run *menu systems*. When you turn the machine on you may find that a menu appears on the screen. This may allow you to type in a choice (a number or letter) to select, for instance, your word processor, database, spreadsheet, graphics and so on.

It works like this. You type in the number (or letter) of your choice. The machine will register that a character has come from the keyboard. It looks in its memory to see if the character corresponds to any of the commands in the operating system. If it does not correspond with any operating system command, it will then look on the disk, in the current directory, to see if this character corresponds to anything which is on the disk. If it finds a file with the character as its first name and a BAT extension for example, (1.BAT), it will associate the character from the keyboard with this particular file. It will open the file and carry out the instructions. These instructions may tell the machine to open the word processor, so it will do this by loading the word processing instructions into the computer's memory. When you exit the word processor you are back in the batch file. The next instruction in the batch file may be to show the menu on the screen. The menu will be re-displayed so that you can make your next choice.

DOS commands

This chapter has so far looked at two of the special files which are part of the computer's starting up instructions. The remainder of the chapter will look at some of the DOS commands which you may need to use. Application packages provide easy to use functions which are then translated into DOS commands by the software itself. However, it is a good idea to understand and be able to use some of the basic DOS commands. This means that you will have a better understanding of the actions you are performing. Some of the DOS commands are not accessible through most software packages, so a knowledge of them will really aid your use of the computer.

Directory commands

You have already seen the use of the TYPE command to look at the contents of two files. This section will look at commands that are used with directories.

There are three actions that you may want to perform with directories. These are CHANGE DIRECTORY, MAKE DIRECTORY and REMOVE DIRECTORY.

Change directory (CD)

To move from one part of the directory tree to another is a bit like navigating in a car. If you want to drive from one city to another there are generally detailed instructions available which will indicate which roads to follow. They may include landmarks at which point you have to change direction and so on. Basically if you are wanting to move around the disk you have to navigate and give explicit instructions so that the computer can move from one place to another. At the moment the prompt C:\> indicates that the computer is looking at the root at the top of the directory tree in C:. The command to change directory is CHDIR or CD for short. It is always a good idea to minimise the amount of typing, so from now on it will be referred to as CD. To change directory and go into the WP directory, at the prompt type

CD WP <ENTER>

Once you have pressed the ENTER key you should see that the prompt on the screen changes so that it says C:\WP>. This has automatically indicated that the current directory is WP. The prompt has changed because of the command prompt PG in the AUTOEXEC.BAT file (p. 46).

To look at the contents of this particular directory type

DIR <ENTER>

The contents of this directory will be displayed on the screen as shown below in Table 3.1. Here you will see that there are some directories and some files in the listing. As well as the AUDIT, ADMIN and BOOK directories (shown in Figure 3.2), there also appears a single dot and a double dot followed by <DIR>. These abbreviations always appear in any directory that you create. The single dot is a shorthand way of denoting the current directory. the double dot (..) directory is information which every directory holds about its parent.

For the directory tree to hang together there has to be some communication between levels. There are two possibilities. Each directory could hold information about directories above or directories below itself. Not all directories have

Table 3.1 Listing of the contents of the WP directory

.		<DIR>	26-01-93	9.15a
..		<DIR>	26-01-93	9.15a
AUDIT		<DIR>	27-01-93	1.15p
ADMIN		<DIR>	28-01-93	11.55a
BOOK		<DIR>	28-01-93	1.05p
CODE	DOC	14555	26-01-93	12.15p
CODE	SSS	33345	26-01-93	2.44p

subdirectories and some directories have many subdirectories: therefore the amount of information that would be held would be very variable depending on the particular directory. However, all directories have one parent directory. This is a much more consistent way of being able to hold the information so that the tree structure will hang together. A byproduct of this information is that it is also a useful shorthand way of moving from one directory to its parent. Instead of having to type in the part of the directory you wish to move type

CD..<ENTER>

You can now move up one level to the parent directory of the current directory. In this case you will see that the prompt changes from A:\WP> back to A:\>.

To move down one level at a time you can use the CD command followed by the name of the directory and repeat this each time you move through the tree. It is possible to change directory so that you move through several levels in one step. To move from the root (\) to the LETTER directory will involve moving through three levels. To do this type

CD WP\ADMIN\LETTER <ENTER>

CD indicates to the machine that you want to change directory. WP is the first destination. The backslash after WP indicates that this is the end of the name of the first destination. It also indicates that the machine must carry on looking at the next level to find the next destination ADMIN. The backslash after ADMIN fulfils the same function. The machine has to look at the next level and find the destination LETTER.

This is a more complicated direction. Instead of directing someone straight to the end of the street, to find their destination you introduce several stages. Go to the end of the street, turn left, first right, second left etc. You are building up slightly more complicated navigation paths, telling the machine where you want to move to. After you have issued a command like this the prompt will change. In this example it will appear as

C:\WP\ADMIN\LETTER>

You can move as many levels down the tree as you wish at any one time. If you wish to return to the root (\) directory there is a short cut that will allow you to do this in one move.

CD\ <ENTER>

This will work from one level right down to the bottom level of your directory tree.

Make directory (MD)

In LETTER you will remember there are subdirectories for each month of the year. You may decide to open a new directory for a new category of letters. You can make the new directory using the command MKDIR or MD for short.

MD STUDENT <ENTER>

There is no indication that anything has happened. By using the DIR command to look at the contents of the directory you should see that at the bottom of the list is a new directory called STUDENT. It has the date and the time it was created. You will see that this is a fairly straightforward and simple way of making a new directory.

Many software packages will not allow you to make new directories within them therefore the directories must be made in advance. Once a directory exists on a disk software will make full use of it. This MD command is one that you may find very useful.

You can actually make a directory from any point in the tree as long as you provide the computer with a detailed path, or navigation instructions, where to put it. For the above example the new directory could have been added from the root using the path detailed below.

MD WP\ADMIN\LETTER\STUDENT <ENTER>

Remove directory (RD)

If there is no longer a need for a directory it can be removed. It is good practice to keep disks tidy and delete unwanted files and directories. This maximises the storage space available on the disk. This process is known as *housekeeping*. Assume that the REFS directory contains a number of references for staff. If you want to remove the directory from the disk you can use the command RMDIR or RD:

RD REFS <ENTER>

will remove the directory. Sometimes you may find that when you try to do this you get an error message as shown below.

Invalid path, not directory or directory not empty.

Use the DIR to confirm that the directory exists and that its name is correct. The last part of this error message, the fact that the directory is not empty, is probably where the problem lies. This is a DOS fail-safe mechanism to make sure you do not delete files which have still got a use. Directories can only be removed if they are empty. This forces you to go into the directory and have a look at the files, thus making a decision about whether you really do want to keep them or not. The next section will show you how to delete the files. Upon the assumption that you have actually deleted the files, you need to go back to the parent directory of the one you want to remove. You cannot remove a current directory. Then use RD and the directory name. By using DIR after this command you should see that the directory has been removed.

Like the make directory (MD) command, it is quite difficult to remove the directories from many software packages. RD is another DOS command which you may find very useful.

Summary of directory commands

The commands we have looked at so far are CD, MD and RD. They are all directory commands, consist of two letters and end in D.

Parameters

You will have noticed that while using these commands you have had to type in the command followed by a space. This is followed by either the specific directory name or the route or path to the directory in which you are interested. The space is vital. If you leave out the space you will get an error message. This is because DOS takes the word before the space and compares it with the commands in the memory. If you were to type CDWP, with no spaces, DOS would look for a command CDWP. It would not find this command and the machine would give you an error message. By saying CD WP the machine understand that CD is the command and it will look for that and then look for the directory WP, as it will know that CD means change directory, and then look for its destination to move into. The WP part of this command is known as the *parameter*. If you read any DOS manuals you will see the word parameter littered throughout. Basically a parameter is a qualifier for the DOS command.

During the conversation everyone uses parameters all the time. If you were given the answer 'Drive' to a question about how to get from one place to another you would be none the wiser. You probably wanted information about the roads you needed to drive on. The information about the roads is the parameter to the command Drive.

Most DOS commands require parameters, or qualifiers. The DIR command will work with no parameter. This is because it assumes that you want to look at the contents of the current directory. The current directory is the *default* parameter. You can use optional parameters with the DIR command. The wildcard characters, discussed on p. 54, are optional parameters for the command.

File commands

File commands allow you to look at, delete, copy and rename files. The commands themselves require parameters. The parameters are the names of the files concerned. Working at the level of the operating system means that you have to be very specific about the files concerned. You have to include all three parts of the file name when referring to them, otherwise the system will not recognise the name of the file.

TYPE

This command is used to look at the contents of a file. The use of this command has already been demonstrated on pp. 43 and 45, when looking at the contents of the two special files CONFIG.SYS and AUTOEXEC.BAT.

TYPE AUTOEXEC.BAT <ENTER>

This command instructs the operating system to display the contents of the file on the screen. Sometimes when you use this command, to look at files that have been prepared in a software package, the screen becomes littered with very strange characters. These can include smiling faces, hearts, clubs, diamonds, beeps and a whole variety of others. This happen because DOS interprets the contents of the files literally. The software packages each have their own dialect, or shorthand way of recording instructions which they can read and understand. DOS cannot and interprets these instruction simply as the characters themselves. Sometimes you will be able to distinguish and recognise some text amongst the rest of the characters.

DELETE (DEL) or ERASE

To delete or erase files from a disk you can use either of these commands, followed by a space and the full name of the file. DELETE shortens to DEL and is therefore quicker to type.

On p. 50 it was mentioned that it is sometimes necessary to delete files. To delete the files in the REFS directory you could use the CD command to move to the directory and then issue the command

DEL JOAN.DOC <ENTER> and then
DEL JIM.DOC <ENTER>

Alternatively you could delete these files from higher up the tree, provided that you indicate the complete path for the machine to find the files in the relevant directory.

Notice that you have to delete files one at a time. If you then type DIR in this particular directory you will see that these files no longer exist. You can then use the RD command to remove the directory. Remember to move from the directory, at least one level up, otherwise you will be unable to remove the directory.

COPY

The COPY command allows you to make an identical copy of a file. These copies can be made within one directory, or the copy can be deposited into another directory. If you are keeping both copies in the same directory they will have to be given different names. You cannot have more than one file with the same name in the same directory. The copy command requires two parameters or two pieces of information. It needs to know the name of the file that you want to make a copy of and the destination and name of the copy.

For instance in the JAN directory is a file NOTE.DOC. You wish to make a copy and put it into the FEB directory. From the LETTER directory type the command

COPY JAN\NOTE.DOC FEB\NOTE.DOC <ENTER>

This instructs the computer to go from the LETTER directory into the JAN directory. Here it will find a file called NOTE.DOC. That is the first parameter. It tells the operating system where to identify the source file. The space indicates that this is the end of the first parameter and the start of the second. The second parameter is FEB\NOTE.DOC. It tells the operating system to copy the file and place it in the FEB directory and call it NOTE.DOC. When you issue this command you should see a message

1 file(s)copied

To check this out you can then to move into the FEB directory and have a look at its contents.

CD FEB <ENTER>
DIR <ENTER>

RENAME (REN)

It is very difficult to think of names for files which accurately describe their content. It may be that you happen upon a name which would describe an existing file. Alternatively the use of a file may change and you may want to change the name to reflect its new use. You can do this using REN for rename. This command, like COPY, also requires two parameters. The first parameter must be the present name or old file name and the second parameter is the new name.

In this directory tree structure there is a file in the subdirectory FEB called FILE.DOC. This name is not very descriptive and you may wish to change it.

REN FILE.DOC BONE.DOC <ENTER>

By issuing a DIR command you will be able to check that the name has been changed.

Summary of file commands

There are four file commands, TYPE, DEL, COPY, REN. Each of these commands requires the name of a file as its parameter. The file name is the full name – the first name, middle name (or full stop) and surname (or extension).

TYPE and DEL require one parameter. TYPE displays the contents of a file on the screen. DEL deletes a file. COPY and REN require two parameters or file names. COPY requires the name of the file to be copied and the destination for the copy. REN requires the old name and the new name for the file in question.

All of these commands can be issued in the relevant directory, or from any part of the tree structure if the appropriate directions are given to the operating system. For instance to delete JOAN.DOC in the subdirectory REFS from the WP directory the command would be

DEL ADMIN\LETTER\REFS\JOAN.DOC <ENTER>

Just a few examples have been presented here of some of the more commonly used DOS commands.

Wildcard characters

There are two characters that can be used to replace other characters in file names. These are called wildcards. They have a function like a joker in a pack of cards, where the one card can be used to represent any other card. The first wildcard is a question mark which can replace a single character in a file name. The second is an asterisk which can replace up to eight characters in a name.

Question mark wildcard (?)

In the DEPT subdirectory of the FINANCE directory (Figure 3.2) you will see that there are different files with different spellings of the name Reid. By moving into this directory the prompt will display

A:\FINANCE\DEPT>

Using the DIR command will show that this directory contains the files REID.DOC, REED.DOC, REINE.DOC and JONES.DOC. If you are interested in a name but cannot remember how it is spelt, use the ? wildcard. By using the DIR command with an optional parameter you can get a listing of a subset of the entries in the directory. DIR alone gives a list of the contents of the directory.

DIR RE?D.DOC <ENTER>

will give a list of all files whose names conform to that pattern. This means that the third letter in the name can be anything. The file name must begin RE and end D.DOC. This command will list REED.DOC and REID.DOC.

Asterisk wildcard (*)

The ? is not a particularly useful wildcard, but may come in handy occasionally. The wildcard which most people use most frequently is *, which is used to replace several characters at once.

In the AUDIT subdirectory of the WP directory there are a variety of files with a number of different extensions (surnames). By moving into this directory the prompt will display

A:\WP\AUDIT>

Using the DIR command in this directory will list the files. You will see that the files have a variety of extensions. If you are interested in the database files only you can use the optional parameter with DIR making use of the * wildcard.

DIR*.DBF <ENTER>

tells the machine only to list the files in the directory that match *.DBF. This means that they can start with any first name but after the . they must have a DBF extension. This command will list ASTHMA.DBF and DIABETIC.DBF. If you were interested in all the files associated with the diabetic audit you might use the wildcard as shown below:

DIR DIABETIC.* or even shorter **DIR D*.*** <ENTER>

This will list all the files whose first name is DIABETIC (or starts with D). The extension is not specified. You will see listed DIABETIC.DOC and DIABETIC.DBF.

The wildcard can also be useful if you want to delete a number of files at once.

DEL *.DOC <ENTER>

instructs the machine to delete all the files in this directory which have the ending DOC. This occurs in one step instead of having to delete them one at a time.

DEL *.* <ENTER>

This instructs the machine to delete every file in the current directory. It does not matter about the first name of the file or the extension. If you issue this command the machine will prompt you and ask

Are you sure? (Y/N)

You will have to type in a Y for yes or N for no, depending whether you are sure or not. It gives you a second chance before you delete all the files in the directory. The * can be used with COPY.

COPY *.* A:

instructs the machine to copy everything in the current directory (*.*) and the second parameter of the command instructs the operating system that the destination of the copies is the A: drive.

Other commands

PRINT

PRINT requires one parameter, the name of the file that you wish to print. It is unlikely that you will need to use this very often as most commercial software packages allow you to print documents very easily.

DATE and TIME

If you type in the word DATE or TIME the current date or time appears on the screen. If they are incorrect you can enter the correct values.

CLS

CLS means clear screen. If your screen is very cluttered you can clear it by typing CLS. The prompt appears at the top of the empty screen.

VOLUME and LABEL

You may have noticed when using DIR that the first line on the screen is

> volume in drive A is

After this will be the name associated with the disk. This name is known as the name, volume or label. It is an easy way of being able to identify a disk. Of course you can always write on a label on the outside of the disk cover, but these labels may get lost, so it is a good idea to label the disk electronically as well. The disk name may also give you a clue about its contents. The command VOL (for volume) will display the name of the disk. The command LABEL will also display the name of the disk and allow you to type in a label. This means you can change the label of a disk if required.

FORMAT

When you buy floppy disks they are not yet formatted. They do not have the tracks and sector arrangement described in Chapter 1. The tracks and sectors have to be laid down within the magnetic material on the disk surface so that the disk can be used by the machine. To do this you need to use the FORMAT command. From the C:\> prompt type

FORMAT A: <ENTER>

The machine will prompt you to put the disk in the disk drive and press any key to continue. It will then format the disk. Formatting wipes information from disks, if they are already formatted. If you have any data on a disk and you ask for it to be reformatted you will lose all the data which is there already.

If your disk is write protected, that is, nothing can be written onto the disk, you will get an error message telling you that the machine cannot format the disk. If you are not certain whether you want to preserve the information on the disk, it is a good idea to check what is on the disk before formatting. Be very careful with the format command because if you format your hard disk you will lose a lot of information.

DISKCOPY

DISKCOPY allows you to copy the entire contents of one disk onto another. The disks have to be the same format. It is only possible if you are going to copy the contents of one type of disk onto another identical type of disk. If you have two disk drives then

DISKCOPY A: B: <ENTER>

will copy the contents of the disk in A onto the disk in B. If you only have one disk drive

DISKCOPY A: A: <ENTER>

will copy the contents of the disk onto another disk using the same drive. In this case the machine will ask you to insert the source disk into the drive and press any key. The machine will read as much from the source as it can into its memory. When the memory is full it will then put another message onto the screen prompting you to put the target disk into the disk drive. It will then write all the information held in its memory onto the target disk. It will repeat this process until it has copied all the information from the one disk to the other.

DOSSHELL

From Version 4.0 of DOS a new command DOSSHELL has been introduced. The command calls a user-friendly interface to DOS. It has a menu structure so that you do not have to remember the actual commands, but can pick them from the menus. There is a built in on-line Help section that can give you help as you are using the system. The DOSSHELL is very like some of the utility programs that are described in Chapter 4. It gives you a user-friendly front end to the operating system. It allows the use of the mouse to make menu choices. DOSSHELL will draw a picture of your directory tree on the screen so that you can look at your electronic filing system. As you become more expert in its use you can customise your shell, change the colours, add your own programs and add in functions or commands that you find particularly useful.

\P switch and MORE

The DIR and TYPE commands display information on the screen. If the information for display is longer than the size of the screen it scrolls round and moves off the top of the screen so fast that it is impossible to read. There are a couple of techniques to prevent this from happening so that you can actually read one page at a time.

DIR/P <ENTER>

This will show you one page or screen of contents at a time. By pressing any key on the keyboard you will then see the next page and so on. This means that you can look at the complete list of files in a directory, even if they take up more than one page. The \P is a switch for the DIR command. It modifies the behaviour of the command. There are a variety of switches for many DOS commands. As you become more familiar with DOS you will learn how to use them.

The \P switch does not work with the TYPE command. You need another technique to slow down the display of long files. To do this type a pipe symbol (the Shift and backslash keys at the same time) ¦ followed by the word MORE. MORE modifies the TYPE command so that the file is displayed one page at a time. If there are more pages to follow the following appears at the foot of the screen

......More......

By pressing any key you can see the next page but it is not possible to move backwards through the file.

The MORE command works with DIR and TYPE and a variety of other DOS commands.

Advanced uses of DOS

There are many other DOS commands that you may find yourself using as you become a more expert user. What has been outlined here are some of the most commonly used commands that will be beneficial to your understanding for using different software packages.

Most of the files that you create will be done within word processors, spreadsheets, databases and other types of software packages. Occasionally you may want to create a file using DOS. For users of DOS with a version number of less than 5.0 you will have to use EDLIN. This is a primitive line editor. You can enter the file, one line at a time. All the commands are single characters. It is very user-unfriendly and worth avoiding if at all possible. From DOS version 5.0 there is a full screen editor called EDIT. It is an unsophisticated word processor. You can see the whole file on the screen at one time and make changes at any point in the file.

There are many handbooks, books and manuals on DOS where you can obtain more information about the commands outlined here and the many others that are available.

Summary

So far we have covered the hardware of the PC and its development. This chapter has described operating systems, specifically DOS, because for any other applications package (software) to run there has to be an operating system present. Figure 3.1 shows this with the arrangement of the different components in a series of shells. At the heart is the hardware, surrounded by the operating system. Further shells are the applications packages that you may wish to use. Chapter 4 discusses the various types of application packages available. The more commonly used packages are then discussed in more detail in the chapters that follow.

Introduction to the software | 4

Outline

There are many different types of software, or *application packages* available. The choice can bewildering and companies make great claims about what their software can do. For the computer novice, the pressure is on. How do you choose the right one for your job?

This chapter will provide a brief guided tour of some of the different types of software package available. The types of package discussed are probably the ones that will be most useful for clinical audit. It will point out some of the factors to bear in mind when deciding what type of package is required. More details on databases, spreadsheets and word processors are given in the following four chapters. Chapter 12 will look at introducing application packages into audit projects.

What is software?

Software has been defined as: 'The stuff that does not make any noise if you drop it on the floor!' Software is the instructions that tell the computer what to do. Without these instructions the computer will do nothing. Every time you see a computer working, from the in-car computer, automatic bank machines to sophisticated database systems, it is the software that is allowing it to work.

The instructions are written in a computer language and translated into a form the computer can understand (binary or machine language). These instructions are generally stored (on disk or tape) and read into the computer memory as required. The instructions are in the form of magnetic signals that represent a series of 1s and 0s. They are not tangible. The instructions themselves are not visualised, it is their result that are seen.

As the software packages have become more sophisticated they have begun to include context sensitive on-line Help systems. On-line means that the Help screens (like pages in a manual) are available while you are using the software, at the touch of a key (usually F1). This can save a lot of time if information can be displayed on screen rather than having to refer back to the manual. The Help systems are generally context-sensitive, which means that the first Help screen to be displayed will relate to the particular action being performed when Help was requested. The Help systems have indexes so that any area of Help can be accessed at any time.

There are many different types of software packages: games, databases, spreadsheets, word processors, statistics, graphics, drawing, communication packages to name a few.

Databases

A database is a collection of related information. It is a computerised card index. Most modern packages are relational databases. This means that the data is arranged in a series of tables. Categories of information are arranged in vertical columns, also called fields. Individual records are arranged in horizontal rows, with data entries for each of the fields. This table-like arrangement makes it easy to look at and/or change information. Each table can have one (or several) key fields. The keys are used to provide a unique identifier for each record so that it can be used to index each entry.

Data is arranged in tables of related information. There can be several different tables (or files) in the database. As long as the different tables have one column in common with another table (preferably a unique identifier), the tables can be linked together. For example you may have one table of information about patients:

PATIENT: patient number, name, address, date of birth, sex
　　　　　where patient number will be unique for each patient.

There may be a second table of information about the patients that you have seen.

EPISODE: patient number, date of consultation, time of appointment, length of consultation.

You may wish to find the names and addresses of the patients seen after a particular date. You can link the two tables in the database via the patient number column. This is the column that occurs in both tables. You would request the names and addresses of the patients seen after, say, 1 January 1993. The machine would search the date of consultation field in the EPISODE table. Every time a date was after that specified (1 January 1993), it would take a note of the patient number. It would then go to the PATIENT table, match up the patient number and retrieve the name and address.

To perform this kind of exercise with a manual system can be very time consuming. It could take days. The answers from the database will be available very rapidly. Apart from the speed with which you can perform these queries another advantage of using a database is that you can combine your data in any way. As you think of new questions to ask you can make much better use of the data available.

There are many different database packages available. Chapters 5 and 6 give more information about the concept of databases.

Spreadsheets

A spreadsheet is a package that will allow you to hold information that may need mathematical calculations performed upon it. The spreadsheet is divided into rows and columns. Each box produced by this grid structure is called a cell. These cells can hold text, dates, numeric values, times and formulae. The formulae direct the software to perform calculations on specified cells.

For instance, you may keep your own records of expenditure. By entering the appropriate formulae the machine can sum up the values in an expenditure column and work out any calculations that you require. As you change figures, or add in further figures the machine will up-date the sums and other calculations automatically. This can save many hours. When done manually all the sums have to be re-calculated if changes are made. This automatic up-date facility means that spreadsheets are very useful for performing 'what if' analyses for preparing future predictions. The ease with which these calculations are carried out means that you can vary many different parameters for your predictions.

There are a wide variety of different spreadsheets available. They all work in basically the same way and Chapter 7 gives more details about the concept of spreadsheets.

Word processors

A word processor is a program for manipulating text. This can be editing, arranging or sorting text. Word processors allow you to personalise standard letters or alter relevant parts of the letter, leaving the rest the same. It takes the best part of the typewriter and avoids the worst elements. Mistakes can be corrected on screen, before printing. Standard documents can be saved. Only variable parts need to be typed in. This can save many hours of work.

The format of the text can be changed very easily. Paragraphs can be aligned at their left or right edges or justified, as in a book. Parts of the text can easily be underlined, made bold or italicised. Subscripts and superscripts can be inserted. The typeface (font) can be changed either in style (Courier, Helvetica etc.), size or both.

Text can be moved around the document, deleted or new text can be inserted at any point. In some cases graphs and pictures can be imported into the document from elsewhere (either a library of pictures or from another package).

There are many different types of word processors available. They all have the same underlying principles and these are discussed in more detail in Chapter 8.

Other packages

Statistics and graphics packages

Statistics packages allow you to input data and will do any one of a number of statistical calculations on the data. Some of the packages will then allow you to represent the data graphically. The graphics capabilities are integrated into the package. With other packages the data has to be saved onto disk or tape and then input into a graphics package for display.

Desktop publishers (DTP)

These packages are like very sophisticated word processors. They generally have a greater range of font styles and sizes available. They allow the easy manipulation of blocks of text so that the layout of documents can be changed very rapidly. The easy manipulation of blocks of text means that the text can be moved around, placed in boxes or curved around imported pictures. The fonts can vary in size to produce characters from a few millimetres to several centimetres high.

Using a desktop publisher means you can produce very professional looking documents without needing to go to a printer.

Games

There is a wide range of games available. Some of these are very sophisticated with very high definition graphics, for instance the flight simulators and golf games. Some may require a very high degree of coordination, like the space invader arcade games. Others are simpler. The screen displays are not so involved and they may require ingenuity, not speed.

Utilities

Utilities are a very diverse group of programs. Some are auxiliary programs that can work alongside main programs. For instance, you may wish to have access to a calculation while using a word processor. The calculator program could be a utility that you can call up while inside the word processor. Alternatively utilities can be fairly large programs that, for instance, allow you to have easy access to the operating system commands, through menu systems so that you do not need to know the commands.

There are two main types of utilities: resident and non-resident programs. *Resident programs* are loaded into memory and are present when running other programs. They are sometimes called TSRs (Terminate and Stay Resident in memory). They are then accessible at all times. These are small programs that allow you to have access to a variety of useful functions. These functions might include notepads, calendars, calculators etc. These can be accessed when using any other software package. The *non-resident programs* are like conventional software packages. They are loaded into memory and used. Upon exit from the utility they are no longer available in memory. They have to be reloaded before they can be used again. Non-resident utilities are often file managers which present a user-friendly front end to allow you to use the DOS commands without having to know them. They have user-friendly screens and menus that are easy to use.

Viruses and anti-virus utilities

A virus is an unwanted computer program that has the ability to replicate itself. It hides itself on disks. It can copy itself from an infected floppy disk onto a hard disk. Once on the hard disk it can copy itself onto any uninfected floppy disks that are used on the machine. These floppies can then infect other machines. The virus may sit 'quiescent' and do nothing for many months. Only upon a trigger (for instance a date like Friday 13th) does it become active. Some viruses do no harm. They can flash message on the screen. Others can do a great deal of damage. They can wipe all the data from a hard disk, or damage files.

There is a group of utilities that check for the presence of viruses on both hard and floppy disks. This can help prevent their transmission to your machine. If you are worried about viruses it is worth using these virus checkers. It also pays to be vigilant about using floppy disks. If you are uncertain of the origin of a disk do not put it into your machine unless you are going to check it for viruses.

Expert systems

Expert systems are programs that aid in decision-making. They are built up on a series of rules, called heuristics or rules of thumb. These rules are gleaned from experts and developed into a series of IF THEN rules. Sometimes these rules can be given numeric weightings. For a given series of incidents the computer will work out outcomes or probabilities for certain situations. The systems are flexible and can 'learn' new rules while in use, building them into the existing frameworks. In circumstances where there are a great many influencing factors they may be very useful to point the user in the right direction. They will not, however, replace the experts themselves.

Communications software

As computers become linked together there is a need to share information between different users. This is discussed in more detail in Chapter 9. There is a whole class of software that is used to allow users to communicate with one another, across the same network and over several different networks, from one part of the globe to another. The ways that computers communicate are very varied and there is a wide variety of communications software available. Some operating systems have communication commands within them. Again, this is discussed further in Chapter 9.

User interfaces

Unfortunately there is very little standardisation between different software packages. Very often the ESCAPE (ESC) and F1 are the only keys that work in the same way. As discussed in Chapter 1 the ESC key can sometimes be used to get out of (escape from) certain functions or situations, although it does not always work. The F1 key is often used to access the on-line Help screens that are available for the different packages. Again this is not universally true.

The original software package for microcomputers were often very difficult to use, especially for people with little or nor computer experience. They took a long time to learn and a very long time to become expert at using. To overcome these difficulties a variety of different user interfaces have been developed. These have to take into account ease of use for novices and shortcuts for experienced users. The ultimate aim is to develop systems that the users find easy to use and enjoy using.

Menu systems

Menus have been developed to aid in the use of the various types of software. These are often shown on the top, or bottom of the screen. The user can pick one of the options from the menu. This generally involves using a specific combination of keys to activate the menu and make the choice.

There may be several levels of menus. The structure of choices can become very complex. Users can find that they have got lost in the branching structures that may result. In these circumstances the ESC key can be very useful.

Graphical user interfaces (GUI)

When using a GUI the user is presented with a number of pictures (icons) on the screen. Each of these icons represents the files, application programs or functions that the user has access to. The user has to point at the relevant icon, using the pointing device or mouse. To activate the icon the user has to click one of the mouse buttons. This allows new users to feel less threatened by the computer and rapidly learn how to use it.

The success of the Apple Macintosh has proved the popularity of the GUI approach. Many competitors have now gone down this avenue. At present Microsoft Windows is enjoying great success. Windows is one of a range of application packages that runs on IBM-compatible machines and allows them to be used like an Apple Macintosh. It is like another layer above the operating system (see Figure 3.2). Application packages communicate with Windows, which in turn communicates with the operating systems, which in turn communicates with the machine.

The GUI desktop

When any GUI is first opened the user will see a number of boxes laid out on the screen, each box having one or more icons (see below) within it. This is known as the desktop. Each of the boxes, known as windows (see below), will be labelled, indicating the functions that it contains. Each icon will also be labelled indicating its exact function.

Using the mouse the user can customise the appearance of the desktop by moving and re-sizing the windows on the desktop. As the application programs, or icons within the windows, are opened they can be regarded as running in their own window on the desktop. These windows can also be moved and re-sized on the desktop. It is therefore possible to have several different programs running at the same time.

Windows allows the user to make greater use of the computer and the pay-off for this is that it requires a certain amount of power from the machine. Although it is possible to run Windows on a 286 machine it requires a 386 chip to work properly. It also requires at least two, but preferably four, megabytes of RAM.

As application packages are designed to communicate with Windows there is a drive to standardise the interfaces. What this means is that the software designers, from many different companies, are now trying to make their packages look and feel like the other packages. The menus are often in the same place, have the same types of options and operations. This means that the learning curve for a new piece of software is dramatically reduced.

Windows, Icons, Mouse and Pulldown menus (WIMP)

Windows Every time you open a new piece of Windows software (spreadsheet, word processor, drawing packages etc.) it appears in its own window. The size of the windows can be altered and several windows can be opened at the same time. This means that there may be several different software packages open at the same time. This is known as multi-tasking. If you want to draw a picture the picture can then be copied into a document created in a word processor. Text produced in the word processor can be copied onto a spreadsheet. This is discussed in more detail in Chapter 9.

Each software package works in its own window, but the information contained in the various files being used in each different package can be transferred. This immediately increases the potential of the computer. Windows or windowing is the generic term used to describe this use of the computer. (It is also used by Microsoft to name a specific application package).

Icons On the screen are various pictures (icons). These include arrows and pictures of buttons on the screen. These icons can be activated with the mouse (see below) or from the keyboard. They have certain functions associated with them. This can be a quick way of activating different functions, without having to go through various complicated menu systems.

Mouse These graphical user interface packages can be used in conjunction with a mouse. The mouse can be used to move some pointing device around the screen. Depending on the software itself, the functions activated at the time or the position of the pointing device on the screen, it will vary in shape. By pointing at the relevant part of the screen, using the mouse, the various functions/commands available can be activated by pressing one of the mouse buttons.

Commonly there are one or two buttons, but sometimes there are three or more. In most packages at present, where there are two buttons it is generally the left button that is used. As the packages become more sophisticated there will be an increasing use of the right hand and other mouse buttons. Mice have been designed to be easy to use. If too many buttons are introduced they will become increasingly complex and this defeats the objective.

One note of caution about using the mouse. The shape of the pointer is very important. Once you get used to a particular package you will recognise what functions are available to you with each pointer shape. Always make sure the pointer is the correct shape otherwise you may not be able to instruct the computer as you expect.

Pulldown menus With menu interfaces the whole of the menu is generally shown on the screen. If you choose one menu item you may then be taken to a subsidiary menu, and so on, until you reach the choice you require. With WIMP interfaces only the name of the menu is shown on the screen. You can activate the menu by using the mouse or keyboard. Once activated, the menu options are listed in a pulldown menu. By activating the choice you want, the function will be performed, or a further dialogue box will appear on the screen. If the dialogue box appears it is because you will have to make further choices about the command before it can be performed.

The function keys and the ALT and CTRL keys in combination with any key from the keyboard often allow short-cut ways to perform the tasks for the more expert user (Chapter 1).

The graphical use interface and WIMP packages can give the user the feeling of being more in control of the computer and are proving to be very popular.

What You See Is What You Get (WYSIWYG).

This is further refinement of the WIMP packages. The screen looks like a piece of paper and text, graphics etc. are arranged on the screen exactly as they will appear on the printed page. This is very helpful to the inexperienced user and can greatly aid the production of professional documents.

Some of the more conventional packages have a coloured screen (sometimes blue or green). As the text is typed it appears on the screen. If some of the text is formatted (e.g. underlined) it appears as a different colour or has some type of marker at the beginning and end of the formatted area. With practice the user does recognise what each colour represents on the printed page. It is more intuitive, however, to see the screen the same as the final print out with the formatted areas actually shown as such. For this reason WYSIWYG packages are becoming more popular.

Multi-media

A new development that involves both hardware and software is the advent of multi-media. This is the integration of video images, stills and sound onto the computer. This will allow segments of sound, or images, to be embedded into other computer applications. This has great potential for educational uses of Information Technology but its impact is likely to be much wider in the future.

The incorporation of these different media requires a lot of the computer. Extra processing power, video and sound cards and other modifications are often required. The images and sounds require enormous amounts of disk space for storage. Techniques are being developed to help reduce the needs, but at present the hardware costs are very high.

Software copyrights

When you buy a piece of software you buy a licence to use it. By its very nature information stored on disk is easy to copy. This leads to the temptation to use pirate copies of the software. This infringes the terms of the licence.

Using software is like reading a book. Only one person can read one particular copy of a book at any one time. If more than one person wants to read the book it has to be photocopied although everyone knows that this is an infringement of copyright. When you buy software your licence allows only one person to use it at any one time. It is possible to get a site licence, so that there are a predetermined number of legal copies within an organisation.

If you are using a network there will be a special licence agreement to allow a predetermined number of people to access the software at the same time.

Software manufacturers have used several different ploys over the years to try to stop piracy or illegal copying and use of the programs. Some software is copy protected. It will allow you to make a certain number of working back-ups. If you try to copy it more often it will self-destruct. This can introduce problems if your disks and back-ups become corrupted as you may be unable to use your own legal software. Another way that manufacturers have tried to protect their software is to use a *dongle*. A dongle is a device supplied with the software that plugs into one of the sockets at the back of the computer. The software checks that the dongle is plugged in before it will operate.

Nowadays most software is not protected, but the first time the software runs it prompts you for a name and serial number. Your name is then stamped on the software. Any pirated copies can be traced to their source.

Shareware and freeware

Some software is produced that is meant to be free, or very cheap. It is often written by enthusiasts who are keen to distribute it. Sometimes there is a request that you register for a nominal sum. This is usually to allow the author to further develop the program. Freeware and shareware are sometimes distributed on free disks that accompany some of the computing magazines. They are also available over bulletin boards. Bulletin boards are areas of common storage where software and messages are stored. Users can access them remotely, by linking in their computer to the relevant networks. Once linked into a bulletin board you can have access to the software that is lodged there.

Summary

This chapter has looked briefly at the commonly used application packages and some of the other types of software that you may come across. It has also outlined the different user interfaces that are available.

The next chapters in this section will look in more detail at the more commonly used types of application packages: databases, spreadsheets and word processors. The final chapter will look at sharing data and resources.

Designing a database | 5

Outline

Data collected for audit comes in all shapes and sizes. It will depend very much on the planned project. There may be numeric data (percentages, test results, ages etc.); textual data (names, addresses, drugs and drug regimens, comments etc.); codes (ICD9, OPCS4, READ etc.); dates (date of birth, admission, discharge, date of last test etc.); true or false (Yes/No) responses to questions. How can these diverse types of data be handled best by the computer?

Generally the type of software best designed to handle a variety of data types is a database. There are very many different databases available on the market. There are software packages that can be bought 'off-the-shelf' and used to make databases for each individual project. At the other extreme there are ready-made packages, often written by specialist companies, or the Information Technology (IT) Department of the Health Board or Health Authority. These may be resource management systems, audit systems, case-mix systems, patient administration systems, GP systems etc.

Owing to lack of knowledge, these databases are sometimes regarded as 'black holes'. There are many cases where departments have collected data and input it into a computer for years – but no one knows how to access it! Obviously in these situations it is a waste of time to put anything into the computer at all.

Databases all have the same underlying principles. They allow users to input data into the computer. This information is stored, manipulated and can be retrieved at a later date (Chapter 6). The majority of modern databases are called *relational databases*. This chapter will cover some basic points about the structure of databases so that you will be better informed, will be able to plan your own databases or get more from your existing systems.

Relational databases

As explained in Chapter 4, a relational database is a collection of data conceptualised as a series of tables. Each table is composed of rows and columns.

Each row is known as a record and contains information in each column. Each column is also known as a field. The first step in designing a database is to decide what information is required. When a commercial company is supplying the software this may be done in conjunction with their development team. Having prepared a list of the information that you require, this data will have to be pulled together into related groups. These groups will form the basis of the tables.

Before looking at the tables, consider how the computer reads and searches through information. The memory of the computer is limited. Very large tables of information may not 'fit' in the memory. To overcome this, the computer will 'juggle' the data. It will hold some data in its memory. When it looks at another part of the table, the first part, already in memory, will be lost. The next part of the table overwrites the previous contents of the memory. This goes on until the computer has looked at, searched, the whole table.

Because of the memory limitations it is a good rule to try to make the tables as narrow as possible. The narrower the table the more likely that each complete row can be held in memory at the same time. This allows the computer to search for the data in the table more efficiently. What this means to you, the user, is that information is found more quickly. This can be likened to a table published in a book. If the columns of the table extend over more than one page, especially if the reader has to turn the page to continue looking at the information, it is difficult to keep track of the information. If the table is narrow enough to fit on one page, but the rows extend over several pages, it is still relatively easy to read.

Database design

The whole point about using a database is that the stored information should be accessed very easily. The database should be arranged to make looking at the data, and making any changes, as straightforward as possible.

Key fields

You can define *key fields* (or indexes) for your tables. Keys have to be unique. If you decide *Patient number* is going to be a key field then the machine will not allow two patients to have the same number. Another advantage of having indexed tables is that information stored in the table can be retrieved more quickly. To return to the book analogy, trying to search for a subject in a book without an index takes much longer than using a book with an index.

In a table there can be more than one field within the key. In the DEPENDANT table shown in Figure 5.1 *Patient num* will be repeated for each dependant of a particular patient. However, the combination of this number with *Dependant name* will be unique. *Doctor No* and *Patient No* form the key in the EPISODE table shown in Figure 5.1. As each doctor sees more than one patient, the combination of the two numbers, or fields, will be unique.

Remove repeating groups

One of the important considerations, as was discussed above, is to keep the tables as narrow as possible. To do this the first step is to look at the tables one at a time. Table 5.1 provides a list of the information for a fictional audit project.

Table 5.1 Data to be collected for audit project

| | List of data items to be collected | |
PATIENT	DOCTOR	EPISODE
Patient	Doctor	Episode
Patient number	Doctor ID	Doctor No
Patient name	Doctor name	Patient No
Patient address	Doctor address	Length of Consultation
Date of Birth	Dept code	Primary diagnosis
Sex	Head of Dept	BP
Dependant name	Location	Smoking status
Dependant age	Grade	
Dependant sex		
Occupation		

The first group of data collected together to form a table is about the PATIENT. There is information about *Patient number*, *Patient name*, *Patient address*, *Date of Birth*, *Sex*, *Dependant name*, *Dependant age*, *Dependant sex* and *Occupation*. Obviously the information collected will depend on your own specific project. The example here is fairly simple to make the point. Within the patient data are some fields for information about dependants. There could be a column for each *Dependant name*. If so, there would have to be enough columns for the maximum number of dependants. This, for the sake of argument, might be 10. Now if the average number of dependants is three there will often be seven empty columns and so on. For the *Dependant age* and *Dependant sex* there will be further empty columns. This is an inefficient use of the computer. How can this be overcome? In the PATIENT table is a column called *Patient number*. This is a unique number that will identify each patient. This column, or field, can also be used in a new table called DEPENDANT (see, for example, Table 6.2). This new table can hold the *Patient num* and have further columns for dependants, *Dependant name*, *Dependant age*, *Dependant sex*, as shown in Figure 5.1.

The two tables have got the *Patient number* column in common; although the column has a different name in each of the tables the data contained in the columns is the same. This common field can be used to link the PATIENT and DEPENDANT tables in order to find out the ages of the dependants of a particular patient. All you have to do is tell the computer that the data in the two columns is the same. If you are looking at patient 007, the computer will search for *Patient num* 007 in the DEPENDANT table and each time it finds an entry for this number it will retrieve the ages of the dependants.

Data independence

In the DOCTOR table the fields for *Head of Dept* and *Location* are independent of the doctor. They depend on the department itself. If all the doctors working in one department were to leave, then the information about the head of department and location would be lost. If the head of department or location of the department were to change, then all the records for all of the doctors would have to be changed. By removing these fields (*Head of Dept* and *Location*) from the DOCTOR table and placing them in a new DEPARTMENT table, along with *Dept code*, and any other details required, departmental data will not be lost when members leave. Also changes to *Head of Dept* and *Location* need to be made only once, in the DEPARTMENT table, not for each record in the DOCTOR table.

The reorganisation of the data into these tables is called *normalisation* (Figure 5.1). The whole idea about producing the database in this form is to allow for minimum redundancy of data (i.e. repeating data items) and to produce the easiest methods for updating and deleting information without losing any data. If data is accidentally lost, due to poor database design, it will have to be re-keyed. This takes up extra time and resources. Normalisation does mean that more tables are produced. However, these tables allow for easier updates and tend to be narrow, which means that they can be searched rapidly.

Each of these tables will be stored as a file and all of the files will relate to one another. Files that do not relate to one another are known as *flat files*. For instance, the data files that are used to input data into a statistics package are flat files.

Information has to be gathered to be input into the database. There are many ways of collecting and entering information, but they are outside the scope of this book.

Data validation

As data items are entered into the computer they can be validated or checked. The software packages can be instructed to look at the data items as they are entered and check that they conform to pre-set rules.

The computer can check that any dates entered are valid. It will not allow 31 September, or 29 February in non-leap years and so on. This is very useful and

PATIENT

Patient number*	Patient name	Patient address	Date of Birth	Sex	Occupation

DEPENDANT

Patient num*	Dependant name*	Dependant sex	Dependant age

DOCTOR

Doctor ID*	Doctor name	Doctor address	Dept code	Grade

DEPARTMENT

Dept code*	Head of Dept	Location

EPISODE

Doctor No*	Patient No*	Length of Consultation	Primary diagnosis	BP	Smoking status

Figure 5.1 Audit data arranged as tables after normalisation. * = Keyed or indexed fields.

can save a lot of time. The checking can be made more subtle. It can prevent you from entering dates of birth after the current date, details relating to episodes before the date of birth, certain birthdays or other relevant dates.

If you are entering the results of a test that, for the sake of argument, always lie between 6 and 15 units, you can make sure that the computer will not accept values of 5 or less or 16 and above. If the result of a test is negative in 90% of cases, you can get the computer to default to negative. This means that the result of the test is automatically entered as negative. If the result is positive you can overwrite the automatic entry with the word positive. This will save a lot of typing when entering the data.

You can set up the database so that as data is entered it can be formatted, to fit a predefined layout. For instance you may wish all patient numbers to have a hyphen (-) after the third digit. By instructing the machine to do this you will not have to type the hyphen each time, it can be automatically output. This predefined layout is called a picture and is also commonly used in spreadsheets. It is discussed in more detail in Chapter 7.

Other types of checking may be to check that no male patients are diagnosed as pregnant, no females have prostate operations, no children have Alzheimer's disease and so on.

The level of validation, or checking, will depend on your needs. The more people who are using the database, you may find the greater the need for validation. Building some of the more complex or subtle validation checks into a system can be time consuming. It may well be that you have to compromise with a certain level of automatic checking. Data validation is discussed again in Chapter 12.

Although the computer can do a lot of the validation for you this does not ensure that the data entered are correct. The data might be in the right range, with a valid date, a recognised code etc., but they may not be correct for the particular patient. For instance, to go back to the test results which are always between 6 and 15 units. The value of 10 will be accepted by the computer even if the correct value for the particular patient is 14.

The saying 'Garbage In Garbage Out' (GIGO) is very important to bear in mind. You may be able to enter any data you want into the database, but if it is not correct, then the answers to your questions or queries will be worthless. The computer can do as much validation as is required but you, the user, have to be sure that what you are entering is correct and relevant.

Summary

This chapter has described some of the features of database design. It is worth looking at the ways to maximise the use of the computer when designing databases. The next chapter looks at some of the ways in which data can be retrieved once stored in a database.

Querying a database | 6

Outline

The previous chapter described how to set up a database to hold data. This chapter will explore the ways in which that data can be retrieved. It will look at the principles involved when asking questions of any database system. It will then discuss the different ways available to display the results of the questions as reports, tables or graphs.

Asking questions

The beauty of using a database is that once the data is stored it can be readily accessed. Any number of data items can be accessed very rapidly. This allows the data to be combined in any way so that previously unexplored relationships can be examined. The same data, stored on paper, is accessible but it can take many hours to retrieve. If more than one item of data is required the time for access can expand exponentially even in the best organised manual systems.

Databases allow you to make maximum use of your data, as it can be accessed in any number of different combinations. You can look at whole data sets, or limited ranges (subsets) of the total data set. This allows very flexible use of the stored data. As far as audit is concerned, the ability to look, rapidly, at certain items of data is a great advantage.

Querying the database

The computer jargon for asking questions of the database is *querying*. Most of the computer-based Clinical Information Systems have a querying option on them.

The actual methods for asking questions vary from database to database. In some cases the reporting facility will already be set up. It is as simple as choosing an option from a menu. At the other extreme it may involve typing in a sentence in a special query language used with that particular database system.

Building queries

Queries can be built up in any system, using the same principles. These principles make use of Boolean algebra, which is based on a binary system of 1s and 0s (true and false).

Boolean logic functions There are three functions that can be used in any order or combination. These functions are AND, OR and NOT. The functions are used in conjunction with a number of comparison operators (see below).

The Boolean logic functions can be described in terms of their *truth tables* (Figure 6.1). For the sake of argument, a 1 represents true and a 0 false. For simplicity, the truth tables show only two parts to a statement or question. The following holds true for any number of component parts to a question.

AND			OR			NOT	
00	0		00	0		0	1
01	0		01	1		1	0
10	0		10	1			
11	1		11	1			

Figure 6.1 Truth tables for AND, OR and NOT.

AND
The answer is false if both halves of the question are false.
The answer is false if one half is false and the other true.
The answer is true if both halves of the question are true.

OR
The answer is false if both halves of the question are false.
The answer is true if one half is false and the other true.
The answer is true if both halves of the question are true.

NOT
Simply reverses the sense, i.e. it changes
true to false and
false to true.

The AND operator will only include any areas of the overlap between the different parts of a question. It is exclusive. The OR operator will sum the two halves of the question. It will include all areas covered by the different parts of the question. It is inclusive. The use of the AND and OR operators is not what you would expect from their English usage. OR is inclusive and AND is exclusive in Boolean logic, the opposition to their meaning in natural language.

AND OR

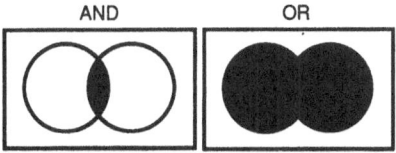

Figure 6.2 Venn diagrams to show the truth tables for the logical functions AND and OR.

Comparison operators The comparison operators are used to build up the questions which the machine will then apply to the database. The answers will be True or False and these answers are then used by the AND, OR or NOT statements.

These comparison operators are:

Equals	=
Not equal	<>
Less than	<
Less than or equal to	<=
Greater than	>
Greater than or equal to	>=

Building questions

To illustrate how you build questions, let us assume that you have a database table PATIENT which includes the patient number, name, address, date of birth and sex of a list of patients, as shown below in Table 6.1. This is the PATIENT table described in Chapter 5, without the occupation column.

Table 6.1 Patient table with some details available

Patient No.	Name	Address	Date of Birth	Sex
1	Tom Jones	1 High Street	14.04.52	M
2	Jean Smith	5 Main Street	23.05.63	F
3	Lucy Tonks	18 Low Street	21.09.50	F
4	Martin Hope	6 High Street	09.10.78	m
5	Bob Green	43 Low Street	31.11.66	m
6	Ann Brown	16 Main Street	12.12.86	F
7	Jack White	24 Lake Street	04.04.73	M
8	Kate Mack	38 Low Street	30.02.88	F

Listing Male Patients – Using OR

If you want to list just the male patients you could ask the database to find all the patients with either 'm' or 'M' in the sex field. Generally these packages distinguish between upper and lower case letters: they are known as case sensitive.

By asking for the names and addresses of the patients where the sex equals M you would get a list of:

Tom Jones

Jack White

By asking for the names and address of the patients where the sex equals m you would get a list of:

Martin Hope

Bob Green

If both upper and lower case forms of the letter have been used to identify the sex in the database you must combine them in the question.

In the example described above, the sex column allows a single entry to denote male or female. The query is aimed at listing all the males who can be denoted by an upper case M or a lower case m. As the M and m are mutually exclusive there will be no overlap between them. AND works by looking for areas of commonality, or overlap, between the expressions in the question. This means that it will not be useful in this context. The OR operator works by including all areas covered by the expressions in the question. It will be useful in this case. By phrasing the question as '●●● where sex equals M or m' the computer will search the sex column and each time it encounters either M or m the answer to the question will be True. The computer will then retrieve the name and address. This means that the complete list of males will be displayed. If there is any other character present, for instance F or f, the answer to the question is False and the computer will not retrieve the name and address.

Listing patients of a defined age range – using AND

To illustrate the use of AND, look back at the PATIENT table above (Table 6.1). Suppose you wish to retrieve the names and addresses of all patients born between 1.1.1960 and 1.1.1970. Dates are stored in the computer as the number of days since a 'zero' date. The 'zero' date is often chosen apparently arbitrarily by the people that designed the system initially. The details need not concern the users, the useful thing is that when dates are held in this form they can be sorted in ascending, or descending chronological order. To look at patients born after 1.1.1960 the question would include:

Date of Birth >= 1.01.60

This will list all patients born from 1.1.1960:

Jean Smith

Martin Hope

Bob Green
Ann Brown
Jack White
Kate Mack

Some of these people are too young for the survey. The second half of the question should be worded to include:

Date of Birth <1.1.1970

This will list all the patients born before 1.1.1970

Tom Jones
Jean Smith
Lucy Tonks
Bob Green

Some of these people are too old for the survey. The survey is interested in the people who appear on both lists, at the overlap of the date ranges. The question halves can be combined to give a question containing the following:

Date of Birth >=1.1.1960 AND Date of Birth <1.1.1970

This will produce a list:

Jean Smith
Bob Green

the people whose birthdays lie in the desired range.

This is a simple example. These functions can be used for more complex questions with many component parts.

So far, the queries have concentrated on looking at subsets of data held in one database table. More often you may want to look at data that is contained in more than one table. In Chapter 5 the example tables PATIENT, DOCTOR, EPISODE and DEPENDANTS were described. The following queries will build on these tables, to describe how to extract data contained in more than one table. The fields in the tables are shown in Table 6.2.

Table 6.2 Database table arrangement after normalisation

PATIENT	DEPENDANT	DOCTOR	DEPARTMENT	EPISODE
Patient number*	Patient num*	Doctor ID*	Dept code*	Doctor No*
Patient name	Dependant name*	Doctor name	Head of Dept	Patient No*
Patient address	Dependant sex	Doctor address	Location	Length of Consultation
Date of Birth	Dependant age	Dept code		Primary diagnosis
Sex		Grade		BP
Occupation				Smoking status

* = Keyed or indexed fields.

Linking tables together

Suppose you want to look at the names and addresses of patients seeing all the doctors who were at a specific clinic over a set time period. The data to answer this question is held in two tables, PATIENT, for name and address, and EPISODE, for the particular doctors. Each doctor, in the EPISODE table, is known by a numeric code or identifier. For the sake of argument assume that you have coded the doctors at the clinic as numbers 3, 7, 12 and 14 (these numbers can be decoded using the *Doctor ID* field in the DOCTOR table).

To link the two tables, PATIENT and EPISODE, the machine must be told that the tables have a column in common. In this case the data held in *Patient number* in the PATIENT table is the same as *Patient No* in the EPISODE table. This is the data element that will be used so the two tables can be linked.

The question will have to include a request to list the names and addresses of the patients who saw one of the doctors (3 OR 7 OR 12 OR 14). Note that in this instance the OR function is being used with more than two components. The wording of the question will depend on the system that you are using, but will be similar to:

List Patient name Patient address where Doctor No = 3 OR 7 OR 12 OR 14
Patient number = Patient No

The machine will search the *Doctor No* column in the EPISODE table. If it finds any one of the four numbers above it will retrieve that patient number. It will then link to the *Patient number* column in the PATIENT table. When it finds its match (the same number) in the *Patient number* column the computer will then retrieve the name and address of that patient.

Increasingly complex queries can be built up from these discrete tables of information. As you become more practised with querying the data your questions will become more and more sophisticated.

Other queries

As well as the types of queries that have been outlined above, most database packages will allow users to do other types of enquiries of the databases. For both alphanumeric and numeric types of data the values in the database can be sorted into ascending or descending order. Inexact matches can be found. This can be very useful. For instance this will allow searching for names where you cannot remember exact spellings or searching on only part of a postcode. Some database will allow searches that seek out particular values and can automatically change them if required – a type of spelling checker!

Numeric queries

As well as the queries described above, numeric data can be manipulated using a variety of mathematical and statistical functions. It is possible to do calculations involving values held in different fields. If the values are in different database tables these tables must be linked (as described above) before the calculations are described. Queries of this sort include multiplying, dividing, summing and subtracting numbers; finding minimum, maximum or average values; using a number of mathematical functions, for instance trigonometry, for calculations. Some of these functions can also be performed on dates. Adding and subtracting dates can be very useful for working out dates of next appointment, times between appointments, ages and so on.

The types of functions described in the above two paragraphs will vary depending on the database being used.

Looking at the results

Reporting

Most databases will retrieve the answers to your questions and produce them in report form. You can design your own reports so that data is presented in a way you find more useful. This may be tabular, or with each field of the record grouped in a particular way, as address labels or a series of test results for instance.

Graphing

It may be most appropriate to view the data graphically. Many databases allow for the automatic production of a variety of different graph types. You can choose the type of graph (pie, bar, histogram etc.) that you feel is most appropriate to the data you have to present.

Exporting to other application packages

Data can also be exported from database packages and used by other types of software. This is discussed more fully in Chapter 9. You can take the data and use it in a statistical or graphical package, if this type of analysis is not performed by the database itself.

Databases and audit

In the ideal situation, with the increasing use of computerised systems, more and more routine data will be collected and stored in databases. In the future audits on this type of data will be relatively straightforward. It will simply be a case of asking the appropriate questions. It will then be possible to repeat audits at predetermined intervals with very little extra work. More planning and effort will be necessary where audit requires the collection of extra data. This is discussed in more detail in Chapter 12.

With the present increasing volume of data and constraints on time, computers will become an indispensable tool in audit. An understanding of the structure and method of interrogating the databases available will be an essential skill for audit. The format of the questions will vary from system to system. It may be as simple as choosing an option from a menu, if the queries and reports have been set up in advance. It may be more complex and require a sentence to be typed in at a command line. In all cases the questions will be based on the principles outlined in this chapter.

Summary

The previous chapter looked at the structure of databases. This chapter has looked at the use of Boolean algebra to retrieve information from a database. It has also discussed a number of other types of queries that are available. As application packages become more powerful they also become more similar. Some of the features of databases, described here, have been incorporated into spreadsheets. These are the subject of the next chapter.

Introduction to spreadsheets | 7

Outline

A spreadsheet is very sophisticated electronic ledger. It is the ideal type of software package to use if you have numeric data, upon which you want to do some calculations.

There are a variety of different spreadsheets available. They all have the same underlying principles and capabilities. This chapter will explain how to start using a spreadsheet, how to enter different types of data and instructions for calculations. It will also describe some of the ways in which you can use the application package to present your results. It will discuss the advantages and disadvantages of using spreadsheets.

Getting started

When you start up the spreadsheet the computer screen will have a grid of rows and columns. Each box in this grid is called a *cell*. The column headings are marked along the top of the grid (usually A–Z then AA–AZ etc.). The row headings are marked along the side of the grid (1–1000 etc.).

Spreadsheets can have a large number of columns and rows. In the majority of cases you will not need very large spreadsheets. As the size of the sheet increases, more memory is needed and if its size exceeds the amount of memory available then the machine can only see part of the sheet at any one time. This means that the manipulations on the data become slower.

Only a small proportion of the spreadsheet will be shown on the screen at any one time. You can scroll (move) around the document to see the rows and columns that are not initially visible. There are different ways to move around the sheet. Some spreadsheets allow you to use a mouse, others do not and you will have to learn the various keyboard commands. This usually involves using the arrow keys. As with word processors, discussed in Chapter 8, it is worth spending some time learning how to move around the spreadsheet.

Different information types

Each cell on a spreadsheet can hold a variety of different information.
1. Data
2. Format Instructions
3. Formulae
4. Notes

Data

This is the numbers (or text) that you have collected and entered. It could be the amount for each credit or debit from an account, dates, times, numbers etc. It could also be headings for columns or rows or commands you wish to add to make the spreadsheet easier to read.

Format instructions

The range of formatting instructions depends on the package being used. Generally they all offer right, left and centre alignment, bold and italic typeface, underlining, shading and a variety of other choices. The format can also 'force' the output to appear in a certain way. This is described on p. 85.

Formulae

To get the machine to do calculations you must be able to input the instructions (formulae) to the relevant cells. This is described below.

Notes

You may wish to attach a comment to a cell. For instance, if you have built up a complete formula you may want to write yourself a note about it. This will be held in the cell, although it will be invisible unless you want to read it. This means that when you come back to the spreadsheet after a few months the note will remind you of the logic used to construct the formula.

Entering data

Each cell on the spreadsheet has a grid reference. The active or current cell is often highlighted. Sometimes it is a different colour, or has a dark outline around it. The *address* (or grid reference) of the active cell is usually indicated on the screen. As you type in the required contents for the cell they will appear adjacent to the grid reference (in some spreadsheets they also appear in the cell). Once you have entered this information it appears in the cell. Make sure that you change the active cell before entering more data. If you do not change the active cell, using one of the commands to move around the sheet, the next item you type in will overwrite the original contents.

The data that you can enter includes the titles for rows and columns, to clarify the purpose of the spreadsheet; comments you wish to add to the spreadsheet; textual data; numeric data. The numeric data can be in several forms. It can be numbers, percentages, currency amounts, dates or times. Provided that you let the machine know what the data represents, you can do a wide variety of mathematical calculations on it.

Some of the latest spreadsheets available are 'intelligent'. If you begin to enter a data series and outline the range of cells into which this series is to be entered the application package will fill in the data for you. All you have to do is enter enough data for the machine to work out the pattern. For instance, if you are entering a column of the dates of each Monday in the financial year, after entering two dates the machine will be able to work out the pattern and fill in the appropriate dates in the rest of the column. If you are entering numeric data which exhibits a pattern (every even number, every third number, the days of the week and so on) the machine will be able to work out the pattern and do the rest. If you are entering only weekdays you will have to enter a full set of the names of the days, excluding Saturday and Sunday by entering a second Monday.

Entering format instructions

You may wish to align numbers or text down the centre of a series of cells. To do this you have to select or block mark the cells you are interested in. In some cases it may be simpler to mark the complete row or column. You can then issue a centre alignment command. Once the machine has received your command you will see the entries re-align as you wished. You can do exactly the same for making items bold, shading cells or a whole variety of other formatting instructions, depending on the particular spreadsheet you are using.

Pictures

For the machine to be able to do any calculations all data has to be entered as dates, times or numbers. There is a conflict when you wish the numbers to have pound signs and commas so that they look like currency amounts. If you type a £ the machine automatically assumes the entry is textual and it will not perform any calculations. Similarly if you type dates, e.g. 2-Feb-93 it will treat the entry as text.

To overcome these problems you can format the cells involved so that the machine automatically overlays these characters onto the numbers you have typed. This also saves a lot of time. If you have to input only the figures you save several key strokes per entry.

You can format numbers to appear any way you like, with any added characters (symbols for different currencies or other characters as required). These formats are sometimes called *pictures*. Each spreadsheet has a list of formats or pictures built into it. You can use these, modify them or make up completely new ones.

Spreadsheets use the hash symbol (#), 0 or 9 to represent numbers in formats. If you use a 0 to represent a number in a format (or picture) you may get some unexpected displays. If the format is larger than the number being input in will be preceded by leading zero's. The format will expand if the number input is larger than the picture. The hash pictures will expand or shrink to accommodate the input numbers. For examples, suppose you decide that the most appropriate format or picture is:

£00,000

this will put a pound sign in front of the number and a comma every three digits from the right.

Inputting 134276121   it will appear as: £134,276,121
Inputting 123   it will appear as: £00,123

This can be overcome by using a picture that includes # to represent numbers.

£##,###

Inputting 134276121   it will appear as: £134,276,121
Inputting 123   it will appear as: £123

Using the zero in your pictures can be very useful if you want to align numbers. For instance £##.00 will cause a column of numbers to align along the decimal point.

£12.31
£16.27
£14.00

Using the same picture with the # symbol instead of 0 after the decimal point – £##.## – will result in the numbers aligning as shown.

£12.31
£16.27
£14

Formats or pictures can be used for numbers, dates, times and percentages. To format text entries the range of formatting instructions will vary between the different spreadsheets, but will generally include underlining, bold, italic, changing font style and size, shading cells and making borders around cells. These formatting instructions are similar to those discussed for word processors (Chapter 8).

Entering formulae

The point of using a spreadsheet is to get it to work out calculations for you: to sum columns, work out percentages, calculate differences between two dates or times or perform any of a wide range of mathematical functions that are available. By using the grid reference for a cell its contents can be incorporated into the formula. For instance, to calculate the sum of numbers entered in cells A5 to A27, you could build up a formula:

sum (A5 to A27)

You can type these cell addresses directly into the formula, or mark out the range of cells required on the spreadsheet. The machine will then automatically enter the grid references into the formula. If you wish to sum a large number of cells, maybe a column of 300 entries, it is quicker to type in the start and end points than to mark them on the spreadsheet. Sometimes the word 'to' in the formula can be replaced by a colon (:), a full stop (.) or two full stops (..) to denote the range of cells involved. The conventions for entries in the formulae will depend on the particular package involved. Each package will have a list of the mathematical functions that it can perform. The functions can be used in conjunction with one another to build up very complex formulae.

Cells that contain a formula will also contain an answer. The answer will be displayed on the screen and may require formatting as described above.

The answer to one formula can be used in another formula. This allows you to build up fairly complex calculations. If your formulae cover a range of cells in a column (for instance A5 to A27) and say eight more rows are added, the range automatically expands to include the new rows (the example would now be A5 to A35).

Entering notes

If you instruct the machine that you wish to enter a note, you can type the text that is required. This text will be attached to the cell, although you will not be able to see it unless you specifically request to read it.

Looking at results

In some cases getting the spreadsheet to analyse data by using a series of calculations is more than sufficient. However in some instances you may require more sophisticated analysis of your data. It is possible to use a spreadsheet to do further analysis on your data once it has been entered.

'What if' analyses

Once the formulae are in place you can change data in the participating cells. The answers to the formulae are automatically adjusted. This makes spreadsheets very useful for 'what if' analyses.

What if we employ another partner?
What if we employ another nurse?

What if the rate of interest changes to X%?
What if we change the number of appointments?

Decide upon the formulae that are required and enter the relevant data. By putting the variable data (salaries of partner and/or nurse, interest rates etc.) into cells the grid references can then be included in the formulae. The variable data can then be changed as often as you like, without having to change the formulae. As these figures change, all the answers to the calculations will also change. This allows instant access to the effects of the proposed changes.

It is always a good idea to put any constants that you wish to use in formulae into cells of their own. For instance the VAT rate can be entered into all the formulae that require it. However, when the rate changes all the formulae have to be altered. This may involve a large amount of work. If the rate is in a cell on the spreadsheet its grid reference can be built into the formulae. A variation in VAT rate involves one change, that of its value in the appropriate cell. This way you can be sure that all the affected formulae will be correct. If you have to change each formula individually it is very easy to overlook one.

Databases

With some of the more modern spreadsheets it is possible to use data that has been entered as a primitive database. A range of cells can be selected from the spreadsheet and the machine instructed that they are to be treated as a database. You can then frame questions, as discussed in Chapter 6, and make enquiries of that data. This can be very useful if, for example, you are looking for all instances of a particular value in the data that you have entered. If you wish to look at another set of data you have to define that set as a new database and the original database is lost.

Once the spreadsheet has done the calculations for you, you will wish to look at the results.

Graphing

It may be enough to look at the figures in tabular form, but numeric data is often best examined in graphical form. Spreadsheets have been designed specifically to look at numeric data, so they generally have excellent graphics associated with them.

The most modern packages offer 64 or more different types of graphs such as pie charts, column charts, line graphs, histograms and 3D graphs. Some even allow log plots. The history of the development of these packages has been for business applications. Their scientific graphing facilities are only now beginning to be developed.

The packages ask you to define the range, or series, of cells that you require to be displayed on the graph. If you have several series these can all be defined and they will all be included on the graph with different colours/patterns for each series. There is then the facility to add legends, text, arrows, titles, axes, labels and so on.

The result looks very professional. These graphs can be drawn on the actual spreadsheet, or separate from it. Because data from the spreadsheet is being shown on the graph the two are linked. In some packages as you change the data on the spreadsheet the graphs will change automatically.

Printing

You can print out a spreadsheet. As with word processors, some spreadsheets have a page preview so that you can see how it will fit on the printed page. In some packages you can instruct the software to fit the spreadsheet onto the whole page, or scale it appropriately so that part of it fits onto a page. You can print the spreadsheet with or without the grid lines and the resulting output will look very well presented. The choice of printer may be important if your spreadsheets are to become official documents. As discussed in Chapter 8, the decisions about what type of printer to use will depend on the quality of output required and the cost. Spreadsheets also require printer driver programs, so that the printer can be instructed correctly (see Chapter 8). Some spreadsheets have the ability to show negative currency amounts in red on the screen. Using a colour printer this can be reproduced on the page.

The graphs can also be printed. With laser printers the output obtained can be of a professional standard. If you have a colour printer you can produce the graphs exactly as they appear on the screen.

Disadvantages of using a spreadsheet

Using a spreadsheet can give you great savings in time and allow you to do some very sophisticated calculations rapidly. However it can take some time to become proficient in its use. The more modern spreadsheets do make this learning curve easier to overcome. There are on-line Help facilities that give help about most of the tasks that you may want to perform. There are often tutorials built into the software, that allow you to work through some exercises at your own speed. The correct answers are provided.

The number of drafts produced may also increase. As you realise the potential of the software you will become more fussy about the way the documents look. The volume of paper that you use may likewise increase.

Another disadvantage is that it is easy to be tempted by the sophisticated calculations available. You may find that you become wrapped up in what the machine can do and end up with something totally meaningless. Increasing the complexity of the calculation is not always the best thing to do. Sometimes simple calculations will give you the most informative answers.

The sophisticated graphics available can be tempting. Some of the graphs that the software can produce look very impressive. However on closer examination they may not be showing your data to best advantage. Do not be tempted to use the 3D graphs when a 2D graph actually tells you more and is less confusing. As with the level of calculations available, often the more simple graphs will give you the most informative answers.

Summary

This chapter has given an outline of the different types of data that can be entered into a spreadsheet, how they can be formatted to give the desired output and how they can be manipulated to do various calculations, including 'what if' analyses and database type enquiries. The graphing capabilities of spreadsheets have been discussed as well as the advantages and disadvantages of using them. The chapter has concentrated on software for handling numeric data, the next chapter describes word processors and their use for handling textual data.

Introduction to word processing

8

Outline

A word processor is a programme for editing, rearranging and storing text. There are many functions that a word processor can perform, some of which are very sophisticated. It is unlikely that any one person will ever need to use all the functions available. Generally, users settle down to a subset of frequently used commands and occasionally employ some of the others. The point to remember here is that the computer is a tool. It can help to produce professional looking documents, or to automate repetitive tasks. If you can do that by using just some ten commands, why worry about all the others which are not useful to you? As you become more expert you will find other commands that may be helpful to you; like learning any application package, it is an evolutionary process.

There is a bewildering array of different word processors available. When these different programs are loaded onto the computer they produce screens that look very different. They do, however, all perform the same basic set of functions. This chapter will describe the sort of things that are possible and the advantages (and disadvantages) of using a word processor over a conventional typewriter.

Getting started

Starting a document is like beginning to write on a new, plain piece of paper. Depending on the word processor that you are using there will be one of a variety of different screens. If you have a WYSIWYG word processor (What You See Is What You Get) the screen looks like a blank piece of paper. As you type the text appears like printing on a page. When the finished document is printed it appears exactly as it did on screen (see Chapter 4). Other word processors have a coloured screen on which the text appears. It does not look like the final printed page.

Somewhere on the screen there will be a menu. It is important to learn how to make the menu choices. This may be done using a mouse, if one is available, or from the keyboard. Introductory manuals for each package or the on-line Help system (Chapter 4) will let you know how to do this. As you become used to the package you will find shortcuts to produce the desired effects.

After finding out how to use the menu commands, one of the most important functions, one which you will need to know how to do right from the start, is to move the cursor around the screen. The cursor is usually a flashing line or box. It indicates where text will appear when you type. If you have a mouse you can use it to move the cursor. If you are using the keyboard, it is often the cursor or arrow keys that you will use. Sometimes it may be a combination of CTRL and arrow or other keys.

The screen often displays information about the status of certain keys. You will notice that there is a key labelled CAPS LOCK on the keyboard. Once this is pressed a light should appear on the keyboard to indicate it is on. All the letters you type will now appear as capitals, although the keys with symbols are unaffected and the Shift key has to be used as described in Chapter 1. To turn CAPS LOCK off you just have to press the key again. It is a toggle: it toggles, or switches, between the on and off states. There are several other toggle keys and their status should be indicated on screen as described below.

If CAPS LOCK is on, the word CAPS will appear, generally along the top or bottom of the screen. There is also a NUM LOCK key. If this is on it allows you to use the numbers from the numeric keypad. If it is off, these keys will act as arrow keys. This will also be indicated on the screen. If NUM LOCK is on the word NUM will appear. There are several other indicators and some of these will be discussed below.

Word wrap

When using a conventional typewriter you are alerted by a bell as you near the end of each line. This allows you to press the carriage return key to start a new line. With a word processor the words you type automatically 'wrap' onto the next line. This is known as *word wrap*. It is very useful as it means you do not have to watch what you are typing on the screen. You only need to press the RETURN/ENTER key to start a new paragraph.

Editing

Inserting text

Once you have typed some text there may be changes required. It is very easy to insert words or sentences within the body of the text. Position the cursor at the point at which you wish to make the insertion and start typing. The existing text will move along to make room for the new text. The machine will automatically cause the new text to word wrap so that the paragraph will remain intact.

If you wish to overtype some of the existing text with new text, you can go into overtype mode. As you type new text it overwrites what was there originally. Using most word processors, to get into overtype mode you have to press the INSERT key. Somewhere on the screen the abbreviation OVR will appear. (Generally this appears near the indicator that lets you know if the CAPS LOCK is on, see above.) This is also a toggle switch; by pressing INSERT again this OVR will disappear. Some word processors display INS when in insert mode (the opposite of overwrite).

Deleting text

Deleting text is also easy to do. As with inserting, you can move the cursor to the word or sentence you wish to delete. If you wish to delete a few letters or a word, you can position the cursor at the start of the text to be deleted and press the DELETE (DEL) key. This will delete characters from the cursor forward. Alternatively you can position on the cursor at the end of the text to be deleted and press the Backspace key. This will delete characters backwards from the cursor. Many word processors have commands so that you can delete text words or lines at a time. If you have a large block of text that you wish to delete from your document you can mark or select that block and press the DELETE key. The whole marked area will disappear. Each word processor has different ways for selecting or marking blocks of text.

Most word processors have an Undelete or Undo command available. If you accidentally delete some text you can often retrieve it. Note, however, that this Undo will only undo the last command issued.

Block commands

One of the most useful features of a word processor is that it allows you to move text around and re-arrange it. This is generally known as Cut and Paste, an analogy from the days when reorganising text meant cutting out sections from paper documents and pasting in the paper at its new location! Using a word processor allows this sort of operation to be done very rapidly.

Delete, Move and Copy If you have a section of text that you wish to move from one area to another you first have to select or mark the block of interest. Once marked, you issue a command to cut out the block. Note, however, that this Cut command is different from the Delete described above. What happens here is that the cut block is stored in an intermediate storage area (sometimes called the *clipboard* or *stack*) so that it can be accessed later. You then move the cursor to the new position for the cut text and issue a Paste command. The cut text will then be pasted in or moved to the new area. Some word processors ask you to mark the block and move to the new position without going through the Cut stage.

If you wish to duplicate some text you can select or mark the block required and issue a Copy command. A copy of the text is then placed in the intermediate storage area. You move the cursor to the new position and issue a Paste command. The text is left in its original position and copied to the new position. You can copy the block as many times as you like. Some word processors will ask you to mark the block and move straight to the new position and will directly copy the marked block, without using an intermediate storage area.

The intermediate storage area will hold the last item that you cut or copied. If you issue a new Cut or Copy command the previous contents are lost.

Search and Replace

Another very useful facility used for editing documents is Search and Replace. You can ask the word processor to search for particular text, either one or more characters, whole words or sentences. You can then instruct the computer to change them or replace them with different characters or text.

For instance, if you realised you had spelt 'thier' instead of 'their' throughout the document you could use Search and Replace: Search for 'thier' and Replace with 'their' throughout. In this instance it will be quicker than doing a spell check (see below).

Formatting

Once text has been entered its appearance and layout can be altered. This can be done at a very local level, changing individual characters, or at paragraph, at page or document level by changing the arrangement of the text on the page.

Character formatting

Each word processor has its own selection of formatting options available. Before you type in text you can choose from these options. The subsequent characters that you type will exhibit the choosen characteristics, or combination of characteristics. Formatting commonly available includes underlining, double underlining, embolden (bold), italic, subscript and superscript. There are usually a number of different fonts (typefaces) available each with their own range of sizes. This means you can have say several typefaces in a range of sizes and italicised, all in one document.

If you have text already typed that you wish to format, you can select or block mark the relevant text and choose the desired formatting characteristics. Only the selected text will be changed. That on either side will remain unaltered.

In a WYSIWYG word processor the formats that you choose will be shown on the screen. This means, for example, that bold text will appear as such on the screen. In other types of word processors the formatted characters will appear a different colour from those around them. With practice you will become familiar with the colour coding. The formatted characteristics will appear as expected on the printed page.

There are some application packages available that supply you with extra fonts. In some cases this software can be loaded onto the computer itself. In other instances it has to be loaded onto the printer. There are font cartridges that can be purchased to enhance the range of fonts available to the printer.

Paragraph formatting

With a conventional typewriter most documents are *left justified*. This means that all the lines are lined up on the left hand margin. For most printed books the text is justified. This means that both the left and right hand margins are lined up. Using a word processor you can choose a variety of paragraph formats – right, left, both ends justified or centre justified. In centre justified text each line starts in the middle of the page. As text is entered it is adjusted so that each line is symmetrical. This can be very useful for centring text.

If you issue a command to produce one type of justification this will be active for all subsequent paragraphs. If you want to change the alignment or justification of one or several paragraphs that you have already entered you will have to select or block mark the relevant paragraphs. Then you can issue the alignment command and the selected text will be altered.

You can also choose whether to indent the first word in a paragraph, so that it is done automatically. You can also choose the line spacing between each paragraph. It is also possible to indent complete paragraphs if required. As you become more used to your own particular word processor you will become aware of all the options available to you.

Page formatting/layout

As well as altering the format of individual characters and paragraphs it is possible to set out commands for page layout. This include setting margins, number of columns on a page, the width of tab stops, how headings are displayed and how to deal with different levels of headings. You can choose to have automatic numbering systems for headings which can indicate subheadings, e.g. 1.0, 1.1, 1.1.1 etc., or you can ask the machine to grade headings automatically. Main headings might be in a larger size of print and bold, with subheadings smaller and underlined etc. You can also set up different levels of indentation for different sections of the document.

There are very many options available in the different word processors. If you find that you use a number of standard letters, once you have decided the layout of these the outlines can be stored as templates. These templates can be called up onto the screen to allow you to fill in the relevant details, without having to retype the standard wordings each time. This can be a great time saver.

Other facilities

Importing

As discussed in Chapter 4, it is possible using some application packages to take graphs, pictures or text produced in one piece of software and import them into documents created in other application packages. Some word processors will allow you to import these diagrams, graphs etc. in this way. You can then structure your text around them.

Text alignment in columns

One problem with word processor is aligning text in columns. Using the space bar to space out characters, numbers or words does not produce the results expected. The columns may appear to be lined up on screen, but when printed they are not. One way around this problem is to use the tab key and predefined tab stops. Each press of the tab key will take the cursor to the next tab stop. The text that appears lined up by this method will be aligned on the printed page.

A sophistication of this method is to use tables. This facility, however, is not available on all word processors. Where it is available it allows you to define the number of columns required. Using the tab key you move between columns. The grid lines of the table appear on the screen, but unless specified, will not be printed out. Tables make the alignment of text more straightforward. It is easier to add extra text lines or columns. If you enter extra text into tab-delimited columns all the previously entered text will be moved out of alignment. This requires extra work to realign.

Spelling checks

There may be a dictionary built into your word processor. It will check all the words that you have typed to see if they match words in the dictionary. If there is no match with a particular word it will tell you and give you a list of suggestions which may be useful to make corrections. You have the facility to add your own words to the dictionary while using it. The various spell checks may use different criteria to suggest words to you, but they all allow you to type in a correction if their suggestions do not include the word you want. They are obviously very useful, but a word of caution is needed on their use. If any word that it checks is in the dictionary it will not throw up an error. There may be words out of context in the document that are correctly spelt. If you have typed 'there' instead of 'their' for example, the spell check will not detect an error. This means you do still have to proof-read your documents.

Thesaurus

This utility can be used to prompt you to choose an appropriate new word for your text. It is often much quicker than having to look up words in a book.

Mail merge

If you wish to sent out a standard but personalised letter you can use the mail merge utility. First prepare a document which contains all the names and addresses. This can be imported from a database mailing list if you have one. Type in the standard letter with special instructions for the machine to fill in the names and addresses. When you issue the merging instruction the letter will be printed with each individual's name and address in the correct position.

Macros

Macros are short sets of instructions for the machine. They are available in most application packages, in one form or another. They are described here for word processors. They can be very useful for allowing you to make shortcuts when using your word processor. For example, if you find that very often, at the start of a document, you type your own home address in a fancy font, you can automate the process by using a macro. To produce a macro you tell the machine to record your key strokes, both the instructions and the text you type.

Once the recorder (a log that the machine writes all the key strokes to) is turned on, you can select the font, size and paragraph alignment, for example centre alignment. Next type in your home address and then change the paragraph alignment, font and size to that normally used for letters and then turn off the macro recorder. The machine will ask you to for a name for this macro. The macro will be saved under the name you give it. The next time you start a new document tell the machine to run the macro. Your home address will now appear at the top of the document. It saves lots of typing: all you have had to do is type the instruction to run the macro and supply its name.

Others

There are many other utilities available, depending on the word processor you use. These include indexing, allowing annotations, footnotes, book marks etc. These are probably the type of functions you will make use of when you are more expert.

Saving

While you are writing your document its contents will be held in Random Access Memory (RAM). If there is a power cut the contents of the memory will be lost. This means that you will lose your document. If you save it the contents of the document will be written to disk. If there is a power cut you will just lose the work since the last save.

Some of the word processors ask at time intervals, that you decide upon, if you wish to save. When you save the file, you tell the machine where the file is to be written on the disk. If directories exist the word processor can use them and save files where you tell it to (Chapter 3). You will be asked to supply a name for the file. This will be between one and eight characters long. The word processor will automatically add the full stop (middle name) and extension (surname) to the file. If you want to save the file in more than one place you can go through the save operation, indicating different paths (Chapter 3) each time. You can also change the name of the file when saving it for a second or subsequent time. The file with your original name (and original contents) will still exist on the disk.

File size

When saving a document, the larger it is the longer it will take to be saved. It is good practice to break large documents into several smaller ones. If there is an area of corruption on a disk and it occurs in the middle of a large file you could potentially lose a lot of data. If the file is divided into smaller portions the amount of data lost will be reduced.

Large files take longer to be read into the computer's memory. As a user you may find that you become frustrated while waiting for the computer to manipulate your file. As a rule of thumb, document files should be no longer than 10 or 15 pages.

Some word processors also allow you to save in a way that the document can then be read by someone else's, different, word processor. You may have the option to save the file in a different format.

Printing

Print preview

Some word processors will allow you to preview the document before you print it. They will show you one or two complete pages on the screen so that you can have an overview of the document with any diagrams or tables in place. This will allow you to adjust the position for page breaks and margins before printing if you are not happy with the look of the document.

Printing and printer drivers

There are commands in the word processor to ask for the document to be printed. The word processor will send the appropriate signals to your printer so that it will proceed smoothly. In the word processor application package there should be a number of small programs called printer drivers. These programs allow the word processor to give the appropriate instructions to the printer. At some point, maybe during the installation of the application package onto your machine, or when you bought your printer, you will have had to tell the word processor what type of printer you have. This allows the word processor to use the correct printer driver. If you change printer you may find the printer comes with a disk and instructions as to how to install its printer driver so that the word processor can use it. Without this program being present the printer will probably not work correctly.

Chapter 1 included some information about different printers. You will choose your printer based on decisions about cost and the quality required. Once set up correctly there should be no problems getting print outs (hard copy) from your word processor.

Disadvantages of word processors

You can see that using a word processor can give you great savings in time and allow you to produce documents of a very high standard. There are some disadvantages, however. First it does take time to become proficient in their use, although the more modern word processors do make this obstacle easier to overcome as there are on-line Help facilities and tutorials.

Another disadvantage can be the number of drafts that you produce. As you realise the full potential of the application package you will reject documents that are not perfect. Letters which would have been more than adequate when produced on a typewriter can easily be corrected using a word processor. This means that the volume of paper used may increase. Whether working with other people or on your own, the temptation can be to carry on amending documents.

Summary

This chapter has given an outline of the major functions that most commercially available word processors can offer. It has explained some of the jargon associated with word processors and discussed some of the advantages and disadvantages of using them.

The next chapter looks at ways that data can be shared as it is unlikely that users will wish to use only one application package and never share data with colleagues.

9 Sharing data and resources

Outline

Computers were originally designed for single large tasks and multiple users (multi-user). Mainframe and minicomputers could handle tasks that were difficult to do manually because they usually involved large numbers of calculations or collating large amounts of data about a single topic: for example, the payroll information for a large company.

Storing and retrieving data from these large databases requires a number of users to be able to enter and retrieve data simultaneously, so aside from the raw power to perform massive number-crunching tasks, mainframes and minicomputers also allowed a number of users to share the same data and programs. Before the introduction of the personal computer, therefore, computing consisted of multiple users using mainframes and minicomputers, performing either massive number crunching, or accessing large databases. Performing other functions such as word processing came a poor second.

When the PC was first introduced, it was designed to provide 'personal' services to individual users. PCs made it easy for individual users to collect their own information, slot it in and out of different types of programs and even carry the information around with them. Unlike mainframes or minicomputers, PCs were designed so that only one person could use the information stored in a PC at any one time, and so that the computer could only do one task at a time. This chapter outlines the importance of data and resource sharing, and discusses how the problems associated with these initial limitations of the PC have been overcome.

The first section of this chapter will discuss the ways in which data can be shared between different application programs on a PC. The second section will outline the way in which the PC can be made to switch quickly from one task to another, to share data resources so that the user is able to transfer constantly updated data between programs. The final section in this chapter will discuss how to combine sharing of both data and resources between a number of computer users in a multi-user computer environment.

Sharing data

One of the rationales for using a computer to perform any task is to reduce the workload of the user. Part of this workload reduction can be achieved by preventing the duplication of effort inherent in re-doing work that has already been done before. Therefore if information is already stored electronically in one computer application, there are huge advantages in being able to transfer it electronically into another application without having to re-key it.

Essentially, there are two forms of data sharing possible. The first way is to cut a 'chunk' of information (a text or data file) from one application and transfer it to another application without retaining a connection which links the two applications. In the following discussion this type of data sharing will be referred to as a *static* data transfer.

The second way of sharing data is to cut a chunk of data from one application program and transfer it to the second application program, but to maintain links between the two applications so that when the data is altered in the first application, the second application is automatically updated. This form of data sharing will be referred to as *dynamic* data sharing.

Dynamic data sharing is usually a much better way of transferring and sharing information. Mainframes and minicomputers are inherently multi-user, multi-tasking machines and therefore they have always been capable of maintaining dynamic links between different users and different applications. These facilities are now becoming more common for the PC.

Transferring static data between application programs on a PC

Transferring static data between different application programs on a PC is a fairly simple task. It can be done without having both programs open simultaneously, therefore, it can be done by a single-user/single-tasking operating system such as DOS. However, it must be remembered that when static data is transferred, the data in the receiving program is not updated if the data in the original program is altered.

This simple transfer of static information can be done between programs on a single computer or between computers. It can be done between similar and dissimilar applications.

Transferring static data between similar applications

As already mentioned, computer users like to reuse the information that has been collected where this is appropriate and possible. Often there is a need to transfer information from a word processor into another word processor, or from one spreadsheet into another. This situation usually arises because of a wish to access information that has already been collected. The following discussion on how this transfer of static data can be accomplished assumes that the data being transferred is either already on the PC's hard disk or on a floppy disk having been copied on to the disk from another PC.

Copying text This situation commonly arises where a user wishes to access text created in another word processing package. For example, two colleagues may be collaborating on a document using different word processors on different PCs. Document files consist of essentially two types of information. There are the actual letters themselves – the 'A's and 'B's, the numbers 0 to 9 and so on. These are the so-called ASCII characters and the way that they are represented does not vary between word processors. Then there are the *control* characters – the characters that determine the style of the text (bold, italic, underlined and so on) and the way the text is displayed on the page – the tabs and justification. It is usually a simple affair to transfer the ASCII text between different word processing packages. However, the control characters vary between different word processors so text imported from one word processor into another is often interspersed with odd symbols which represent the control characters created by the original word processor.

There are two ways round this problem of transferring document files cleanly between word processing application programs. It may be possible to save the original document as a ASCII file only (i.e. without any control characters), so that a file containing only the bare text is transferred. Alternatively, many modern word processors can import text from other word processors by replacing the control characters in the file with control characters appropriate to the receiving word processing package.

If the receiving word processing package still cannot recognise and convert text from the sending word processing package, it is sometimes possible to convert the text by using a separate text conversion program, or when all else fails, there are commercial companies that specialise in converting text from one format to another.

Spreadsheets and databases Copying data files between different commercially available spreadsheets is usually done in a similar fashion to transferring text. When the spreadsheet is saved onto the disk the machine is instructed to translate the control characters to those used by one of the more popular, commercially available, spreadsheets. When the receiving spreadsheet is reading the data it can then translate the control characters from this intermediate, standard, format to those that it understands. Using a commonly used spreadsheet application program's format means that the data can be imported and exported in the correct rows and columns. It is possible to import data into a spreadsheet in simple ASCII format but the data imported in this way is usually packed together into the first column. To split this compressed data back into the different spreadsheet columns it is necessary to perform a special operation (known as *parsing* the data), and this is often not very easy to do automatically.

Importing and exporting database data files is fairly straightforward if all that need to be transferred are tables of data. As with spreadsheets, standard formats can be used. However it is also fairly easy to transfer tables of raw ASCII text between databases as long as both the exporting and importing packages have a common method of identifying the break between the different fields and records – for example, the comma-delimited format. Using this the exporting spreadsheet or database breaks up the data fields in the exported file using commas so the receiving program can distinguish between the fields. If the fields are fixed in length then no breaks need to be identified provided that the sizes of the fixed length fields exported by the first program are the same as the sizes expected by the importing program.

Transferring static data between different types of applications

In the previous discussion the emphasis has been on transferring complete files of data between similar types of applications. However, the situation often arises where the user only wishes to *cut* a small amount of information from another type of application and *paste* it into the application where they are currently working. For example, if a PC user is writing a letter, they may wish to *open* their electronic address book, find a name and address, *copy* it out of the list of addresses and *paste* it into the letter they are writing. If they are writing a report they may have collected a set of relevant figures or created some graphs in their spreadsheet/graphics package which they wish to paste into the word processor that they are using to write the report.

DOS is a single-tasking operating system, and only really capable of running one program at a time. There are two different ways that chunks of data can be transferred from one type of program to another. The first approach has been to develop application programs with the ability to import chunks of data (textual or graphic) exported from other types of programs. The second approach has been the design of application programs that contain several different modules within them. These application programs are known as *integrated packages*.

Using non-integrated packages to transfer static data Most application programs are designed to be stand-alone packages. They are designed primarily as databases, word processors or spreadsheets and so on. However, software vendors have realised that most users often wish to transfer data between different types of programs. For example, as outlined above, a user may well wish to incorporate graphs from their spreadsheet into a word processed document to produce a report.

The ability to transfer small chunks of data from one type of stand-alone package to another depends on the existence of common file formats that can be recognised by all types of programs. Most leading packages are able to import and export small chunks of data between different types of application program using standard file formats, so that, for example, it is quite easy for a PC user to import a graph from their spreadsheet into their word processed document.

However, transferring chunks of static data between different application programs can be a very time consuming process. The way this is usually done is to open up the *sending* application program to identify, copy, name and save the correct chunk of data within the sending program and then to close it down. Finally the *receiving* application program has to be opened and the saved chunk of data called up (usually by remembering its name) and inserted into the correct place.

Integrated packages

To combat this necessity to open and close DOS based application programs in order to transfer chunks of data, many application programs have rudimentary features of other types of programs built into them. For example, some word processing programs can contain the lists of names and addresses which can be stored and inserted into documents at will.

There are many DOS based integrated packages on the market. They usually contain core modules of word processor, database and spreadsheet/graphics, and many of them contain additional modules such as communication software, clocks, calendars, calculators and so on. The great strength of these types of packages is that as the modules are all designed to work together it is therefore easy to transfer data between them. Some of these packages can even exchange data between the modules dynamically, so that, for example, if a range of cells is created in the spreadsheet module and copied into a document in the word processing module, figures in the word processed document will change if they are altered in the spreadsheet.

Buying an integrated package is often a cheap way to get a number of different programs for the cost of a single one. The major disadvantage of these types of packages is that each of the modules within an integrated package can be fairly limited, and not have the same range of functions that a dedicated stand-alone package might have. The other disadvantage of these programs is that the separate modules are not industry standards, unlike those of the big selling stand-alone packages, and therefore the user interfaces can be fairly idiosyncratic.

An introduction to multi-tasking

If a PC is to be used as a personal tool, to allow the user to work most effectively it must be easy for the user to share data and resources between a number of applications. The user should also have immediate access to the information – after all, no sensible person would swap a paper-based information system such as a diary and address book for an electronic one, unless it gave them an advantage in speed or convenience. There is little point in keeping diary information on a computer unless it is possible to open the diary in the middle of doing something else. If, for example, a colleague rings to find out whether you are free for a meeting on Thursday while you are in the middle of writing a report, it is advantageous to be able to open up your electronic diary without closing down the word processor. These requirements mean that the PC should first be able to switch quickly between one application program or task and another, and secondly it must also allow the user to transfer data between programs with ease. The ability to open more than one program at a time either to access or share information is known as multi-tasking.

If the advantages of being able to switch quickly between application programs are obvious, so are the advantages of being able to transfer data dynamically between application programs. Using the dynamic transfer of data, if the data from a spreadsheet is pasted into a word-processed document, when the spreadsheet data is altered, the document is automatically updated. The ideal working arrangement is, therefore, to be able to open a number of application programs at the same time and to create dynamic links between them so that data transferred from one application program to another can be automatically updated as required. The first section of this chapter has outlined how static data can be shared between application programs. This next section discusses how the original limitations of DOS were overcome to allow for multi-tasking and dynamic data sharing to take place.

Multi-tasking with DOS

Due to the way that DOS uses the memory of the computer (Chapter 2), it is difficult to get DOS to run more than one program at a time. To overcome this, various technical tricks have been devised so that data and resource sharing can take place.

TSRs

TSR (Terminate and Stay Resident) programs, or memory resident programs, are small application programs designed to sit permanently in the first megabyte of RAM alongside other larger programs. They have been discussed in Chapter 4. The advantage of being memory resident is that they can be called up at any time while using larger programs by hitting a predefined key or set of keys (which are known as *hot* keys). Calling a TSR can be done without shutting the larger program down. Some TSRs can be used as *clipboards*. Clipboards are utility programs which can hold small amounts of information, allowing the user to copy a chunk of data from a program while it is running, and paste it into a completely separate program.

The disadvantage of TSRs is that they have to be small and they take up some of the first megabyte of conventional memory and crowd the other programs. They can be badly behaved and interfere with the running of larger programs.

Enhancing DOS

One of the enhancements of the later versions of DOS (such as DOS 5) is a technique known as task-switching. This allows the user quick access to a number of programs at almost the same time. Using task-switching, the user can freeze the current application program by pressing certain predefined keys and jump to another program without having to fully close down the first one. However, task-switching is not true multi-tasking because if a user switches out of a database where a search is taking place or out of a spreadsheet where a calculation is taking place, that task simply goes into suspended animation. In a true multi-tasking situation if a user leaves a program while it is actively completing a task that task will continue while the user is working with a second program. There are a number of memory managers on the market, that work with DOS to allow the user to copy data and switch quickly between application programs.

Multi-tasking systems

DOS is essentially a single-tasking operating system and it cannot easily run two application programs simultaneously in memory. In order to be able to open more than one program at a time, so that data can be transferred dynamically, and to use a PC's resources most effectively, a multi-tasking operating system is required. Although various types of multi-tasking operating system have been developed for the PC, the only two multi-tasking systems which are in common use are Windows from Microsoft and OS/2 operating system from IBM.

Windows

Using Windows to open more than one application program

The graphical user interface of Windows can make it much easier for a novice PC user to open up application programs, and to manage their data files (Chapter 4). One of the major advantages of using Windows over DOS alone is the ability to run more than one program at a time. With the multi-tasking abilities of Windows, portions of CPU time and chunks of RAM can be allocated to different application programs allowing them to be run simultaneously.

The typical Windows session will show the icons of the graphical user interface (usually known as the Windows desktop). The user can start the word processor by pointing to and then clicking on the relevant icon using the mouse. While using the word processor it is possible to open up another application program, such as a spreadsheet. By returning to the Windows desktop the spreadsheet can be started by pointing to and clicking on its icon. These two application programs will then run side by side, the user switching between them at will.

Copying data between Windows application programs

One of the main reasons for opening two different application programs simultaneously is to allow the transfer of data between them. This is done by using the Windows clipboard. This is an intermediate storage area that is used to store data copied from one application before it is inserted into another application. Using the Copy command in the first application program (known as the *server* application), and the Paste command in the second application program (known as the *client* application), the data can be transferred invisibly between the application programs via the Windows clipboard.

Maintaining dynamic links (DDE and OLE) Using Copy and Paste via the clipboard makes it easy to copy static data between open application programs, but Windows allows the user to create dynamic links between application programs using a process known as DDE or *dynamic data exchange*. The method is similar to using the Copy and Paste commands as outlined above, but instead of using the Paste command in the client application program, the Paste Link command is used. This not only copies the data but creates a link between the application programs so that changes in the server application program data are automatically communicated to the data held in the client application program.

With the latest versions of Windows it is possible to go one better and use a method of linking application programs called OLE or *object linking and embedding*. Using OLE to transfer data chunks (or 'objects') between application programs means that when the transferred data is embedded in the client application program, to alter the data object it is not even necessary to open up the application program from which the data came. Merely clicking on the data object in the client application program causes a modified version of the server application program to be opened up with the data object in place ready for editing.

Using Windows to share resources

Another advantage of working within a multi-tasking environment such as Windows is that as well as sharing data, other computer resources can also be shared. This is particularly useful in the area of printing. Windows contains a utility called Print Manager, a spooler, which runs as a background process. Control of the PC can be returned to the user while a printing job runs in the background.

Windows also allows information about the PC peripherals to be held centrally so that a number of application programs can access the information. In previous chapters the use of device drivers such as printer drivers was discussed. With DOS application programs a separate printer driver must be installed on the hard disk for each application program that uses a printer. This causes additional work for the user as well as taking up space on the hard disk. In contrast, when a new

Windows application program is installed, the application program is able to use the printer drivers already installed as part of Windows itself.

OS/2

The multi-tasking features of Windows can also be provided by any multi-user operating system. OS/2 is able to provide similar multi-tasking facilities, but its use as a PC multi-user operating system will not be covered in such detail because at present it is not so commonly used. One reason for OS/2's limited appeal in the field of health care is that running OS/2 demands a lot more technical expertise.

Towards a totally multi-tasking and multi-user environment

It must be said that DOS still remains the most commonly used PC operating system, and that many application programs are not yet fully Windows- or OS/2-compatible (particularly in terms of dynamic data exchange). There is no doubt that as hardware prices plummet and software vendors produce Windows and OS/2 versions of their application programs, the move towards multi-tasking operating systems on the PC will continue.

The prime advantage of multi-tasking is the ability to switch quickly between application programs and the ability to facilitate data transfer between application programs. However, sharing data between different users is even more important in an area such as health care. The final section of this chapter will concentrate on how computers including PCs can be linked to each other or to a mainframe or minicomputer to allow the passage of data between users. Only by allowing multi-user access to health care data will computer systems reach their full potential to aid processing of information about medical care.

The discussion of the topic of multi-user technology will not be as extensive as the discussion on multi-tasking, however, as much of the hardware and software manipulation needed to link computers together requires specialist expertise. Although it is useful for the enthusiastic amateur to understand the basic concepts of multi-user technology, in most situations they will definitely need to rely on trained professional staff to implement multi-user computer systems. The following discussion will therefore concentrate on explaining the basic concepts only.

Multi-user systems

There are important advantages inherent in being able to link users together in any setting. In the first place it can be useful for the sharing of resources, for if computer users are linked together, they can share computer software such as application programs, as well as hardware equipment such as printers. However, probably the most useful function of a multi-user computer system is the ability to share data between users.

There are many instances where the sharing of data can be useful, from the ability to access other users' word processed documents, to the ability to share information stored in a database. As with the discussion on sharing data and resources on a single computer, access to data and resources on multiple computers can be considered in terms of sharing static or dynamic data. Multi-user access is usually taken to mean access to dynamically changing data. However, in order to make clear the distinction between static and dynamic data in this context, the sharing of static data will be considered first.

Sharing static data

Sharing static data is the most basic way to share data between computers. This sort of data sharing is most commonly done by using floppy disks, tapes or file transfer facilities. Sharing static data is fairly easy because there is no need to maintain dynamic links between the original data and the copy. For example, if a file is copied from one computer to another via a floppy disk and the copy is installed immediately on the second computer the information in both the original and the copied files is identical. However, once either of the files is revised, the two versions start to diverge because changes to one file will not be reflected in the second file. Using straightforward copying of files, therefore, is only really helpful when files are being backed up (to provide a copy if the original computer's data storage fails) or to provide copies of data to a number of users where the original data is only used as an initial starting point or as a reference by the new user.

Backing up to floppy disk and tapes, and using file transfer facilities are very similar. Information is being transferred between computers but it is not being shared dynamically. For this reason it is usually fairly easy to transfer files between different types of computer. There are many software file transfer utilities available that allow this. This type of transfer would typically involve a large mainframe or a minicomputer (host computer) running a multi-user operating system and a PC, where the PC is able to access the host computer and download data from it over telephone lines.

A good example of this processing is using a PC to access data or medical reference information held at a distance on large computers. A user will link their PC to the faraway database on a host computer using a modem. The PC will then essentially become a terminal to the host computer. Using database search facilities available on the distant computer or their own PC, the user can then identify the required information on the host PC which can then be downloaded onto their PC for further examination and analysis. Once the data is copied, any changes made to it, either on the host computer or the local PC, will not be communicated. If the information on the host computer is updated, the copied information on the user's PC will not be.

Sharing dynamic data

Sharing static data can be very useful, but it is fairly obvious that multi-user and dynamic use of centrally stored information has many more advantages, largely because any changes in the information are automatically communicated to all users. For example, consider a computerised laboratory system in a hospital. The system will usually contain details on all the tests that have been done. In a big and busy hospital laboratory there will be many different tests being done simultaneously, often at different sites in the laboratory. The ideal laboratory computer system must ensure that all the output from the tests is updated frequently, and the results are simultaneously available at all sites. With the laboratory database held on a computer running a multi-user operating system, once a test is completed, the results can be accessed immediately at a number of terminals all over the hospital site.

Protecting multi-user computer systems

If the advantage of a multi-user computing environment is that a number of users can have access to the data in a number of sites, by the same token maintaining the stability and security of the computer system becomes much more difficult. There are many ways to protect and maintain data on a multi-user system.

Restricting access to data

At the most basic level, users can be given a password. If the passwords are changed regularly and kept secret, unauthorised access to the system should largely be prevented. Within a multi-user computing environment, the users of the computer are usually also divided into different groups and given different permissions. This means that although users can view, alter and delete the files that they have created, they can only view and alter other users' files if given permission to do so. Even if a number of users have legitimate access, to be able to alter the same file, it is obviously essential to prevent them from trying to do so simultaneously. Multi-user operating systems therefore employ a system of record locking, which allows many users to view the file at the same time, while ensuring that only one user at a time can alter it.

Maintaining the data on a multi-user system

On a single-user system a user is likely to feel responsible for performing regular back-ups of the data, for it is only they who suffer if the hard disk becomes damaged and their stored data becomes corrupted. On multi-user systems there is also a need to perform regular back-ups of files held on the computer's hard disk, but as the hard disk will contain information belonging to all the users, it is usual to give the responsibility of performing back-ups to a nominated individual – usually designated the *system manager*. As well as performing system back-ups, the system manager has enhanced powers so that they can add new users to the system, add and change passwords and privileges and generally tidy and maintain the computer system.

Using PCs in a multi-user environment

Obtaining multi-user access to data on a mainframe or a minicomputer is not difficult because mainframes and minicomputers run operating systems such as Unix that are inherently multi-user and have commands that provide for these functions. However, this entire chapter has concentrated on how the PC technology has been enhanced to give PC users similar advantages to users of mainframes and minicomputers. The ability to use a PC as a terminal to a mainframe or a minicomputer in order to access static information has already been mentioned. It is also possible to reduce a PC to the status of a completely dumb terminal to a mainframe or a minicomputer, where it become part of a mainframe and minicomputer system but in the process it loses most of its own processing power (this is known as *terminal emulation*).

PC networks

Although DOS is essentially a single-user operating system, it is also possible to link PCs running DOS in such a way that they can act as a group, sharing data and application programs between them in a dynamic manner. The term *PC network* is used to describe a number of PCs linked together in such a way. PC networks can be set up within a single site, such as within one building. In this situation the network is known as LAN (local area network). PCs networks can also be set up over large distances and in this situation the PCs may be connected via telephone cables or even satellite links. Networks that link PCs over large distances are called WANs (wide area networks).

Networks are essentially created by adding additional hardware components (known as *cards*) to spare expansion slots within the PC itself, linking the PCs with special cables or radio wave links, and running additional software (network software) on top of the PC's operating system. At this point it is appropriate to reiterate what was stated at the start of this section. Setting up and configuring PC networks at present is a very complex affair, and any endeavours in this field are the province of the technically adept. Once the various ways of setting up a network become standardised this situation may well change, and it may be possible for the competent amateur to master the skills more easily. Until this time the best advice to any novice user wishing to set up a network is to bring in an expert.

Summary

This chapter, which is the concluding chapter of the first part of the book, has drawn on the information given in previous chapters on the basics of computer hardware, software and operating systems to outline the benefits of sharing data and resources, first between different application programs, and secondly between different users.

The second part of the book will represent a change of emphasis. By outlining the use of computers in the process of clinical audit, it will concentrate on putting the information that has already been covered into practice.

PART TWO

Putting It Into Practice

Part Two will concentrate on putting the knowledge of computers and software gained in Part One into the practice of audit.

Chapter 10 Looks at the principles of audit, with the emphasis on practical ways to overcome some of the pitfalls.
Chapter 11 Covers the basics of clinical coding, with emphasis on Read Codes.
Chapter 12 Brings everything together in a discussion on how to choose and implement a computer based audit system.

<table>
<tr><td>

Introduction to clinical audit

</td><td>

10

</td></tr>
</table>

Outline

There is no doubt that audit is a buzz-word in the NHS today. There is a large literature on audit itself and the Bibliography at the end of the book lists some of the sources that we have found useful. Most of these publications have not considered the use of computers as a tool to aid audit in anything other than a very cursory way. As the use of computers in audit is increasing, this book has been conceived as a response to the demand for more information on this topic, information which, our experiences have shown, has not previously been available in an accessible format. This chapter looks at the theoretical basis of audit from the authors' viewpoint.

What is audit?

Audit is often divided into *clinical* and *medical* audit. We have used the word audit to encompass both medical and clinical audit. The government's definition of audit, from the White Paper *Working for Patients* of 1989 is as follows:

the systematic and critical analysis of Medical Care, including procedures used for the diagnosis and treatment and the use of resources and the resulting outcome and quality of life for the patient.

In a recent publication funded by the National Health Service in Scotland, entitled *Moving to Audit* (1992), the following definitions are quoted:

taking note of what is done, learning from it and changing if necessary;

improving the quality of care through standard setting, peer review, implementation of change and re-evaluation;

looking at what is done with a view to arriving at acceptable guide-lines and evaluating the outcome.

We think of audit as a way of examining what is going on in health care, in order to answer the basic question:

Are we doing what we are doing in the best way that we can?

Audit interfaces with research and also with the need for management information. A lot of time and energy has been spent disputing the boundaries of these activities. They are different but there are large areas of overlap. In particular there is much confusion about the difference between research and audit. Simply put, *research* is about discovering the right thing to do whereas *audit* is about ensuring that the right thing is done. Audit, research and management information can be used to improve the quality and delivery of health care. Very often the divisions between these activities have been reinforced by funding arrangements.

Why now?

There are several reasons why the topic of audit has gained prominence recently.

1. There has been a general shift to expected accountability from all professional groups, not just health care workers. This has been coupled with a realisation, in all professions, that this activity will be undertaken by outsiders if it is not generated from within the profession.
2. It is becoming increasingly necessary because of the three conflicting forces on health care:
   (i)   limited resources;
   (ii) increasing need and demand;
   (iii) increasing technological advances in diagnosis and treatment.
3. Performing audit is more possible now because of the rapid advances in hardware and software technology.

What are the benefits of audit?

Most health professionals have been doing some form of audit for years, but not calling it that. The purpose of audit is to improve the effectiveness and efficiency of clinical care. It is a tool that can be used to help improve problem areas of work.

Audit can be very educational. Everyone has perceptions about their work, but quite often these perceptions are very different from what is actually happening. By encouraging detailed thought about particular areas of work, audit can lead to a better quality of care. Audit can allow resources (staff, time, equipment) to be maximised by identifying areas where these are used inefficiently. Audit, by giving the detailed knowledge about what is actually happening in a chosen area, can increase bargaining power for new or additional resources. It can help communications, promoting dialogue across all levels and disciplines, and thus aid the process of working as a team.

What to audit?

Generally the audit of health care is traditionally divided into three main constituents: Structure, Process and Outcome. In many cases, however, it may be difficult to split an audit into these constituent parts. Very often the outcome of one audit can be the process of another. The three categories can be defined in more detail as follows.

Structure

This represents the more rigid qualities of health care, such as the staffing levels, buildings, provision of specialised equipment, availability of beds etc.

Process

Process represents the activity undertaken by those involved in health care. For example, examination of the process of health care might look at one or more of the following: the number of consultations, the items recorded in the notes, the frequency of use of particular instruments, the number and type of referrals, the frequency and types of drugs used or investigations ordered.

Outcome

Outcome represents the results of the care given. Although the outcome of clinical care is perhaps the most important area to audit, it is notoriously difficult to measure. For example, it is very difficult to measure the effectiveness of a treatment, because so many factors can influence the outcome. Outcomes can often only be measured after many years of treatment. Another difficulty is that there are very few objective measures of outcome. However, there are some measures that can be used to look at outcomes. These include mortality, incidence of adverse events, health indices and severity ratings, clinical events and patient satisfaction.

Any audit can look at one or more of these areas and it is not always possible to separate them out. In general, when starting audit it is probably easiest to measure structure or process. These are less difficult areas to work in and as you become more confident with the audit methodology you may move onto outcome audits. A common trap that people fall into, however, is thinking that it is only the outcome audits that can improve the quality of care. Very often a systematic investigation of the structure and process of clinical care can have dramatic effects on the patient's well-being.

How to audit?

Audit is usually represented as a cyclical process described as the *audit cycle*, although more recently it has been called a spiral. This is to indicate that, having completed the loop, the starting position for the next loop represents an advance on the original starting position.

The audit cycle

The main points of the audit cycle can be discussed by looking at each stage in turn.

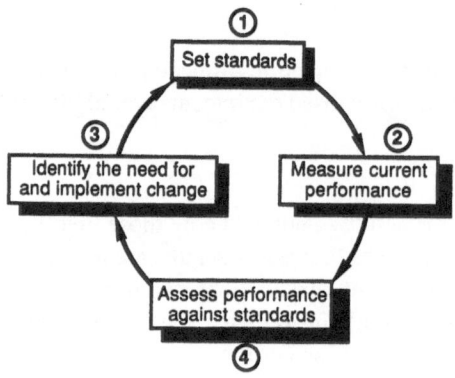

Figure 10.1 The audit cycle.

Standard setting

To *set standards* the first step is to define what should be achieved. In many areas of clinical care there will have to be negotiation with colleagues to get agreement as to what constitutes an achievable standard, bearing in mind local conditions. It can be very difficult to obtain consensus. It is important to distinguish between criterion-based and outcome-based standards.

To produce criterion-based standards there has to be initial agreement as to what constitutes indicators of good clinical care. These criteria should be made explicit and measurable. Outcome indicators are often subjective measures, therefore it can be more difficult to reach agreement. In both situations someone needs to set the standards. It is important to decide who this should be.

1. You and your colleagues When deciding upon standards it is important to bear in mind the particular circumstances that prevail. Standards should be achievable and agreed by those involved so it may be easier to set them locally. However, in many cases there will be at least as many ideas as there are people involved in the discussion! It is important to remember that if the standards set are too ambitious, it is easy for all the participants to become discouraged.

2. You and the profession In some situations there are moves to produce national standards, usually in conjunction with experts in the field. Compared with setting local standards this may initially make it easier to set standards.

However, this method can have drawbacks because local circumstances may make it difficult to use such standards.

3. Outsiders The setting of standards in conjunction with outsiders may be appropriate in some circumstances. However, there is a chance that standards developed in these circumstances can be unrealistic and impossible to achieve. Outsiders may be concerned with features that are irrelevant to the actual improvement of patient care.

Measuring current performance

The next stage in the audit cycle/spiral is to *measure the current performance*. This will require the collection of specified data which must be done in an objective way so that something meaningful will be achieved. The methods used for data collection must be repeatable because audit requires that the cycle is repeated more than once to monitor the effects of any changes. It is at this stage of the cycle that the use of computers can be considered. This subject is covered in Chapter 12.

Assessing performance against standards

Once the standards have been set and the required data collected, the next stage is to *assess the performance* against the standards set. To do this the data collected in stage 2 has to be analysed and interpreted. Along with setting standards, it is often a good idea to define the type of analyses that will be done before starting on the audit. This confers two advantages: first it becomes a natural progression to move from the data collection stage to the assessment stage without having to think about what analyses are to be done. As data collection is generally the easiest part of the audit, it is easy to fall into the trap of not analysing the data, but to carry on instead with data collection. The second benefit of this strategy is that deciding on the analyses first identifies the necessary data items for collection in stage 2.

The next problem that arises is the need to determine who is to assess the data collected against the standards set. If this is done by the team initiating and carrying out the audit, rather than outsiders, there are less likely to be worries about misinterpretation of the results. If the individuals involved in the audit make the decisions about the sort of changes that are necessary, they are also more likely to be achievable. The feeling of ownership may also give everyone a vested interest in ensuring that the changes are put in place and work. It is important to recognise, however, that there may be problems if some of the team are still unwilling to accept that changes may be needed.

If an external body is involved in assessing the results of the audit it may induce anxiety within the team. It can lead to worries about individuals being singled out which can be threatening and impede the progress of the audit. If an outsider is introducing change it may be that the changes are unworkable.

Changes have to be introduced sympathetically because only those people doing the job will have the full understanding of the possible avenues of change open to them. Without outsider involvement on the other hand it may not be easy to persuade recalcitrant members of the team to change their practice.

Implementing change

The results of the previous stages of the audit cycle/spiral are likely to show a need for change. Implementing change is probably the most difficult stage in the audit cycle, for a number of reasons.

First there may be resistance among the auditors themselves, or their colleagues. Most people do not like change or criticism. If anyone concerned in the audit is going to have to change the way in which they work, the discussion will have to be handled sensitively. However, if everyone has been able to have their own say, and been instrumental in the decisions about the types of changes that are required, hopefully there will be a feeling of ownership of the project and the changes introduced will be successful. No audit is done in a vacuum and there may be individuals peripheral to the group whose work will also be affected by the proposed change.

Secondly, expanding on this last point, sometimes the results of a study will show that the solution to the problem is remote or outwith the control of the audit team. In these cases it is possible that the results of the audit may be valuable in providing evidence for necessary changes to those concerned even if they were not originally involved.

Thirdly, there may be no resources available to solve the problem identified. However, in such cases the audit may not have been done in vain because the data obtained may be useful in providing evidence for any subsequent changes.

Finally, having done the audit it is possible that no obvious beneficial change can be identified. In this situation it may be that several cycles of this audit may be required before a workable change is decided upon.

Practical use of the audit cycle

The theoretical model outlined above may not be especially useful in a practical situation. It may not be desirable to start at stage 1 (setting standards) of the cycle; it may, in fact, be preferable to start at some other point in the cycle, or even move between the stages in a different order.

Many of the points raised in the discussion above can be drawn into a checklist. The points listed below overlap with one another and are not presented in any particular order. Some of them are picked up again in Chapter 12, where the practicalities of installing computerised audit systems are discussed.

Practical hints for designing an audit

1   Choose a subject that you are interested in

No one can sustain an interest in a project where the subject under examination bores them completely.

2   Define what you are going to audit

If you do not define exactly what your audit question is, then you may find that you collect a series of data items that will not be very useful. It is generally a waste of time to look at a set of data, collected with no planning, and try to make something useful out of it. Some of the most successful audits, or those which take up little time, have been posed as simple questions. The design of the project has then been focused around answering the question.

3   Get the consent of everyone concerned

If you do not get the consent of everyone you may find that there is no enthusiasm for introducing changes. Generally people require a feeling of ownership or participation of a project before they will help with the process required for the audit. If there is a feeling of ownership it is likely that those involved in the data collection will be more responsible for it and this will help with the validation of the data collected. This will help you to avoid the Garbage In Garbage Out syndrome (discussed in Chapters 5 and 12). Finally, if there is a feeling of participation those involved are more likely to embrace any changes to working practice.

4   Set constraints on data collection

Set aside a certain amount of time for the project. If a reasonably rare condition is under study the audit may run for a long period of time. For common conditions it may be useful to limit the audit to a number of cases, rather than a time period, to avoid collecting too much data. It is all too easy to carry on with data collection, once the data set has been decided; it takes a lot of discipline to stop and analyse the results.

5   Choose a sensible topic

Make sure that the people and equipment available are sufficient for the workload. Do not let anyone overcommit themselves to the project. If they are unable to meet the commitment the project may not succeed.

6   Keep It Short and Simple (KISS)

Do not become overambitious. Make sure that the topic you have chosen can be tackled with the resources (time and people) available.

7   Least Amount of Work (LAW)

Plan the audit so that everyone concerned can cope with the work involved. Everyone will be very busy with their other work. They will only be interested in participating if the extra work is kept to a minimum.

8   Tap into other people's experience

Do not re-invent the wheel. Find out if anyone has done a similar study. If they have maybe they will help you by warning you about any pitfalls they encountered. Maybe they have already designed data collection forms that will be appropriate for your use. If someone else has collected similar data, do you have to do the audit at all? Can you use their data instead?

9   Plan the audit carefully

If you have planned carefully from the start you should have an idea about the questions your audit is going to answer. Do not collect a load of data and start to look through it hoping something useful will result. Do not change your topic mid way through the project. If you do this then you will have different data sets and you may not be able to get anything meaningful from either of them. If new ideas occur to you, set them up as your next audit project.

10   Be underambitious at the start

Do simple audits to start with so that you can build up your skills and confidence in the methods that you are using. Once you are more comfortable with the methods you will be able to progress to more complicated studies. Do not   set your standards too high. If you do not achieve them you may become demoralised. Make sure that the project can be completed by the staff in the time available. If you are overambitious the project may fail.

11   Integrate data collection into routine work

Make sure you know what data you wish to collect. Try to design the data set so that it can be collected as part of the routine work. If this is impossible try to make sure that it can be collected as quickly as possible.

12   Make the data collection forms as simple as possible

If the forms are clear the time taken for them to be completed will be reduced. It may be very difficult to decide upon minimum data sets, but collecting extra, unnecessary, information will increase the time required to do the audit with no extra benefit.

13 Decide on the analysis beforehand

During the initial planning decide what analysis you are going to perform on the data. Analyses can range from complicated statistical tests to simple graphs. Having decided on the analysis beforehand you are unlikely to leave out any important items at your data collection stage.

14 Give clear instructions to anyone involved in data collection

If more than one person is going to be collecting the data they all need to have clear instructions so that the collection will be standardised.

15 Make use of pilot studies

If you have the time and resources it is worth running a small pilot study to make sure that the methods you have devised will work. Sometimes there are unforeseen problems which mean that a particular way of working is impossible: often there is no prior warning that this will be the case. A pilot study will rapidly show whether the methods are workable, whether the data collection forms are usable, whether the right data is being collected and whether the analysis chosen will show the results in a meaningful way.

16 Make sure that all interested parties will be able to look at the results

If the results are not made generally available to those involved there may be some resistance to any changes that are to be made.

17 Be ready to change if the results suggest this is necessary

Remember, if you are not prepared to make changes, there is no point in carrying out the audit in the first place.

Summary

This chapter has presented our own personal understanding of what audit entails. We have looked at why audit has gained so much prominence lately and what benefits it may confer. We have looked at the classical representation of audit as the structure, process and outcome of health care. The audit cycle has been discussed and each stage looked at in more detail. Finally we have given a list of tips that we have found useful when designing a variety of different audit projects.

The next chapter in this section will discuss the principles of clinical coding which are central to the collection of accurate data in any audit project. The final chapter in the book will look at the design and implementation of computerised audit systems.

11

Codes in clinical audit

Outline

A code is a sequence of symbols used in place of a name to identify an object or a concept. Humans do not think well in codes, but computer systems rely on them, particularly in the design and implementation of databases. This chapter will outline the absolute necessity of understanding the use of codes in the management of clinical data for anyone intending to undertake clinical audit.

The chapter commences with a brief discussion of codes and classification systems. It then outlines the use of codes in any computer database to collect, validate, analyse and link data. There is a discussion of the clinical coding systems currently in use (with particular emphasis on the Read Clinical Classification, or RCC, system). The chapter concludes with a discussion of the advantages of using unique patient identification number codes to link patient records across the whole health care system.

Codes and classification systems

From the earliest times, people have felt the urge to order the disparate objects and attributes of the environment around them. This has usually taken the form of first identifying each discrete entity with a name or code, and secondly classifying each entity according to a system of categories. Most children at one time or another have identified an object belonging to them with a listing such as 'this book belongs to Jane Brown, 14 Rose Crescent, Motherwell, Scotland, Great Britain, Europe, the World, the Universe' and so on. This rubric assumes a unique identifier for each entity (name, street address, town and so on) but also a system of classification. The child lives in the street, which is in the town and so on. A coding system only needs to have a unique code for every different object or occurrence that is coded. The allocation of codes to a number of objects can be done on a random basis as long as each object is given a unique code.

To work properly all large coding systems must have an element of classification. For example, telephone numbers are merely unique codes that represent the location of each phone outlet. It would be quite possible to assign phone numbers across the country in a random fashion, or to assign them in order of when they were installed. However, it is much more useful to assign phone numbers by location, so that looking at the first digits of a phone number will tell the enquirer in which town that phone is sited, and looking at the next set of digits is likely to indicate in which area of the town the phone is located.

In general there should be a logic to the way that objects are classified within a coding system if at all possible. When the numbers of objects in a category are small this is not so important. However, where many objects or entities are being coded, a logical classification system is essential.

Using codes in a patient database

The use of codes is an essential part of the organisation and management of any computer database. The basics of using key fields (which are merely codes) in the construction and analysis of relational databases have already been discussed in Chapters 5 and 6. Building on what has previously been covered, the following section outlines in more detail the practical use of codes in a clinical database to minimise the re-entry of standard information, to validate data entry, to keep the database up-to-date and to facilitate analysis of the collected information. It is stressed that although examples from a clinical database will be used, codes can be used in any sort of database to perform these basic functions.

Using codes to minimise the re-entry of standard information

Codes can be used to speed up the entry of recurring data into any database. A code consisting of a single character, or a number of characters can be typed in the place of a longer item of text each time that item needs to be entered. Using the example of a hypothetical computerised clinical database, consider the entry of data on a new patient admitted into a hospital for the first time.

In this situation some of the information, such as the patient's name and address and date of birth, will be entered into the clinical database as free text. However, for the fields where there are only a limited number of categories to choose from, the items are very likely to be coded. For example, when entering the patient's sex, typing 'f' into a sex field may well bring up the whole word 'female', whereas typing 'm' will bring up 'male'. In a similar fashion codes can be used for marital status and type of admission (emergency, routine and so on).

In these situations, a code is being used to substitute a single item of information for each code. However, a code can also link to a number of related data items in a database. For example, in a clinical database, a code can be allocated to each hospital staff member. Each individual staff member's code will be linked to a number of pieces of information on that individual, such as their full name, their title, rank and address.

Returning to our clinical database example: on admission, the patient will be assigned to the care of a particular hospital consultant. When the appropriate consultant's staff code is added to the patient's record, all the information that the clinical database holds on that consultant is linked to that patient's record. Therefore, when the database is required to output any information on the patient, such as the discharge letter, any relevant information on the consultant (such as their name, and their full title) can be inserted automatically into the letter without retyping the information. In the same way staff codes can be used in the clinical database to insert the name and address of the patient's GP.

Using codes to validate data collection

Another major advantage of using codes in any database is that the use of codes reduces the chance of entering inaccurate information. In many situations there are only a limited number of valid choices for any data item. Using our example above, it is unlikely that the patient's sex should be recorded in the clinical database as anything other than female or male. It is sensible therefore to ensure that the only choices the database will accept in this field are 'm' or 'f'. This restriction can easily be enforced by using a coded field with only two valid codes.

In this situation these two codes alone will not be sufficient, because in most circumstances where data is being recorded there will be occasions where the information on any item (be it coded or non-coded) is not available. In general, it is advisable not to leave coded fields blank, and therefore in any clinical database a distinct code should always be available to indicate that the status of a particular item is unknown.

As well as ensuring that only valid choices can be made, the use of codes also prevents different terms being entered for the same entity, such as different spellings for the same item or person. In our example, if a staff member's full details are coded, they need only be entered into the database once (as their details are being linked to their staff code), which means that the details will always appear spelt in exactly the same manner.

Using codes to keep the database up-to-date

A further advantage of using coded items in a database is that it is easy to update information. Returning to our example on staff codes, it has already been indicated that in our clinical database there will be a table of information somewhere in the database where the details of all staff members will be held. The table will have a name, such as STAFF. For each row in the table there will be a unique key consisting of the staff member's code, and a number of other fields containing other details such as their full name, rank and address. When a staff member's details are linked to a patient's details (for example, when details of the patient's GP or consultant are recorded with their admission details) only the staff member's code is stored in the patient's details. The code is used as a pointer to the staff member's full details in the STAFF table.

Imagine the situation if details on any member of staff change – for example if a GP moves practice. If GP's details are always linked to patient records in the clinical database by using the GP's code, it is necessary only to update the GP's address details in the STAFF table. Wherever that GP's code has been stored (for example in any of the database's patient records) the GP code will now *point* to the corrected details. Thus, with the alteration of just one record, all the letters sent to that GP in the future about any patient will be sent to the correct address. This data independence has been covered in more detail in Chapter 5.

Using codes to facilitate data analysis

As well as making the entry of data more easy, and keeping the database up-to-date, the use of codes can maximise the accuracy of data analysis. When analysing a database, if a search is conducted using coded information rather than free text, it is much more likely to bring up all the relevant records. For example, imagine the effect on the clinical database if the consultant's or GP's name in the patient's record was entered as free text rather than by using a code. If the staff member's name had been misspelt in a particular patient's record, then for any search of the full database done using the staff member's name, there would be a good chance that that particular patient's record would not be retrieved. If, on the other hand, a staff code had been used in the database instead, a search using the staff code should identify every relevant patient record.

Using codes to speed up the retrieval by indexing

Using codes can also allow data to be indexed. Indexing data as it is entered into the database can help to speed up its retrieval (Chapter 5). For example, if a search is carried out on a database to provide a list of all male patients, the search can be speeded up if the sex field is indexed. Indexing does have a slight disadvantage, because using an index can slightly delay the entry of data and requires more storage space. One solution in this situation is to enter the data without indexing it, and then index it later at a time when the computer is relatively idle.

Using clinical codes and classification systems

The previous discussion has outlined the use of codes in the collection and analysis of data in a patient database, but the topics covered pertain to the collection of data for any database. The sort of data that has been considered up to now (names, addresses, gender) is likely to be collected in any situation where a database is being used. However, in a clinical database there will almost certainly also be the need to collect data on the patient's diagnoses and treatments. Although this sort of clinical information can be collected as free text, the use of codes provides many advantages.

Clinical coding and classification systems have been in existence for many years, long before the introduction of computer databases. At present there is a wide variety of coding and classification systems for clinical data in use. These coding and classification systems vary from those that have been designed for the use of a particular specialty in a particular locality, to those that are intended to be used in all specialties in all locations. As this book is designed as a introductory text it is not appropriate to cover the details of more than one coding system in detail. Up to now, the most commonly used coding system for diagnostic data in the United Kingdom has probably been the *ICD9* (International Classification of Diseases version 9) in association with *OPCS4* (the Office of Population Censuses and Surveys Classification of Operative Procedures version 4). However, the Read Clinical Classification system (RCC) is rapidly becoming the accepted standard coding system in many areas.

The history of the Read Clinical Classification system

Prior to the introduction of the RCC there was no coding and classification system that was specifically designed to be used in computerised clinical databases. The ICD coding system had already been used for many years for the manual coding of diagnoses in patient records and discharge summaries. Unfortunately the ICD coding system does not provide codes for surgical operations, so other coding operative systems such as OPCS4 have to be used in conjunction with ICD9.

The Read Clinical Classification system is a comprehensive hierarchical coding system designed specifically with computers in mind. It was devised by James Read, a general practitioner, and first introduced in 1983. The first version of RCC was designed solely for use in general practice, and it consisted of a four-digit set of unique codes each linked to a 30-character description known as the Read Code term. Because the RCC was developed just as it became technically feasible and affordable for general practitioners and hospital doctors to introduce computers into their practice, interest in using the RCC spread rapidly, first among GPs and then into hospital medicine.

As the initial trickle of users began increasing, it became obvious that the RCC had the capacity to provide a suitable coding system for many of the computerised patient data systems in the Health Service. In 1990 the RCC became Crown Copyright and Read became the full-time director of the NHS Centre for Coding and Classification based at Loughborough. The NHS Centre for Coding and Classification is responsible for the maintenance of RCC and for introducing new codes. A semi-commercial organisation known as CAMS is responsible for licensing the codes, both to users within the NHS and also to commercial computerised audit system software developers. Because of the way that RCC developed there are several sets currently in use. The NHS Centre for Coding and Classification and CAMS are now working together to convert all RCC uses to the latest revision of the RCC, which is currently version 2.

The format of the RCC

In design the RCC is based heavily on previous coding systems such as ICD9 and OPCS4. However, unlike these previous coding systems, which are held in written form, the RCC exists only as a medical dictionary on a computer file. Because it was designed to overcome the limitations of previous coding systems, the RCC provides a very comprehensive list of codes. Therefore the RCC can usually code any condition to a finer level of detail than the ICD9/OPCS4 coding systems.

The ultimate aim of the RCC is to allow a complete clinical record to be stored entirely in code. For this reason it is designed to provide a code for every thing that a Health Service might need to record about a patient. The RCC is divided into a number of chapters. Chapters 1 to 6 cover occupations, history (symptoms), examination (signs), diagnostic and preventative procedures. Chapter 7 covers operative procedures, and Chapters 8 and 9 cover other therapeutic procedures and administration. Chapters A to T cover diseases (so that, for example, Chapter A covers infectious diseases and chapter B covers neoplasms and so on). Chapters a to v cover drugs. It is apparent, therefore, that if a new entity comes along (such as a new treatment or disease), because of the design of the coding system, a new code for the entity can be identified and allocated to the correct part of the correct chapter.

The components of the RCC consist of, first, the codes themselves (which are structured into a five-level hierarchy, with the detail increasing from left to right), secondly the medical terms associated with the codes, and thirdly the keys and synonyms linked to the codes. Version 2 of the RCC currently contains 100 000 separate codes linked to 150 000 synonyms. Table 11.1 shows an example from the Read Codes, and demonstrates the successive level of detail that can be obtained by adding additional characters to each chapter heading.

Although Table 11.1 shows each of the Read Codes linked to a single term in the latest version of the RCC, each Read Code is linked to one or more terms. The reason that there are often several terms of varying length for each Read Code is that using longer terms prevents the need to use shortened words (such as using 'infarct' instead of 'infarction' for example).

The use of such shortened words has often made the terms difficult to understand. Shortened words also affect the ways that codes can be searched for. However, as computer systems have grown in sophistication, it has become easier for them to deal with longer and longer terms. The NHS Centre for Coding and Classification has taken advantage of this, so that as well as the standard 30-character term, for many of the codes, version 2 of the RCC also provides a more detailed 60- and a 198-character term.

Table 11.1 Examples of Read Codes

Term	Read Code	ICD9-CM
Circulatory system diseases	G....	390–459
Ischaemic heart disease	G3...	410–414
Acute myocardial infarction	G30..	410
Anterior myocardial infarct	G301.	410.1
Acute anteroseptal infarct	G3011	410.1

Using the RCC as a common language

The advantages of using any clinical coding system such as the RCC is that, in theory at least, it creates a standard language which then allows all the different individuals in the Health Service to communicate with each other. For example, the Read Code 'G30..' is used to indicate 'acute myocardial infarction'. If doctor A and doctor B (or manager A and manager B) wish to compare notes on patients with a diagnosis of acute myocardial infarction, they can search their databases for patients with a Read Code diagnosis of G30.. and be sure they are comparing like with like.

The RCC is also designed to work in conjunction with other coding systems. To a casual observer, it may seem that once a choice of coding systems is made for any clinical database, the decision is set in stone because of the difficulties that would be involved in changing from one coding system to another. This is not the case, for as long as each individual code in a coding systems can be linked to a code in another coding system, the actual re-coding of data from one system to the other can be accomplished automatically. Using the RCC as an initial coding system does not therefore preclude the later re-coding of the data into ICD9 and OPCS4 codes.

Converting between the two coding systems is not completely straight-forward. For example, it is impossible to convert from RCC to ICD9 or OPCS4 where there are no ICD9 or OPCS4 codes available. For example, it is not possible to convert Read Codes from Chapter 1 (which covers the recording of occupations) to ICD9 codes, because the recording of occupation is an area not covered by the ICD9 codes. Conversely, converting from ICD9 or OPCS4 to the RCC is not usually problematic because the RCC is more comprehensive.

Problems in using the RCC

There are certain problems inherent in using any large clinical coding system, such as the RCC. First, in any coding system it is obviously a subjective matter to decide what constitutes a discrete and identifiable entity, and to determine where the entity belongs within the coding hierarchy. Secondly, there will always be difficulties in providing a coding system that is large enough to remain comprehensive, without losing the ability to search through it easily. Thirdly, it is often not a simple matter to ensure that any coding system is able to provide the flexibility of using locally defined codes, while ensuring that the codes remain universally applicable.

The difficulties in classifying entities within the Read Codes

There are particular difficulties fitting some clinical specialties into the hierarchical structure. For example, within the RCC chapters, the coding tends to be done on an anatomical basis. This arrangement is more suitable for some of the chapters, as with Chapter B (neoplasms), for example, because neoplastic growths have nearly always been classified by the site of occurrence. However, this arrangement is less suitable for other conditions such as diabetes or endocrine diseases, for example, which can affect many different parts of the body. Within any particular specialty the clinicians may not always agree as to how the disease and treatment entities should be classified.

One of the main problems of designing and maintaining any coding system is the difficulties in balancing the needs of the users with the requirement to maintain the codes as a common language. The RCC was designed as a common method of communication. For this reason, many users find that their own way of classifying and coding does not fit neatly into the framework provided by the RCC.

There is always a tremendous temptation for local users in a specialty to build their own coding system within the Read Code by creating new codes. As well as providing Chapters 1 to 9 and A to v (which are fixed and must not be altered by the users), the RCC also provides two other chapter headings. The @ Chapter is the designated place in which local codes can be stored, and the Z Chapter is reserved for the storage of temporary codes. Although helpful to the local user, the overuse of Z and @ codes in every specialty will eventually undermine the overriding purpose of the RCC – that of providing a common language. Therefore although it is irksome for the users, if they wish to add a new code to the Read Code system it is best to do this in conjunction with the NHS Centre for Coding and Classification. It is up to the NHS Centre for Coding and Classification and the relevant Royal College Specialty Group to decide whether any new code is necessary, and if it is, to then make it available to all users by converting from a Z code to a code from one of the RCC defined chapters.

The difficulties of using RCC in a computerised audit system

A further problem in using the RCC is that there are over 100 000 codes available. Although the coding hierarchy is designed to be as logical as possible it is obviously difficult to find the correct code quickly and easily. The RCC file provided by the NHS Centre for Coding and Classification consists of the Read Codes, terms, synonyms and keys only. It is therefore up to the designers of the computerised audit system using the Codes to create a method of searching through them. In many computerised audit systems such search routines commence with the coder typing in the most relevant part of the term that they can identify. This section of text is used to search through all the terms in the RCC so that all the relevant matching terms can be identified.

This method of searching the Read Code database using only the terms creates problems, because many of the Read Code text fields contain abbreviated words. For example, imagine if the coder is searching through the Read Code terms for the words 'myocardial infarction'. If he or she types in a short text string such as 'infarct', then the search will return many possibilities. If on the other hand the entire words 'myocardial infarction' are typed, if either of the words 'myocardial' or 'infarction' has been shortened in order to fit them into the term, then the search routine will draw a blank.

To try to make the search routines easier, as well as being linked to terms, many Read Code terms are linked to synonyms or keys. For example the Read Code G30.. is linked to the keys 'myocardial' and 'infarction' and the synonyms 'heart' and 'attack'. Therefore, whether the coder types in 'heart' or 'attack' or 'myocardial' or 'infarction' the correct code will be identified. Providing keys and synonyms in the RCC is a way of trying to guess what the average coder will do. In the case of myocardial infarction, the synonyms and keys that the average coder is likely to choose are fairly obvious but there are many situations where this is not the case.

The problems of using a limited list of RCC

Because of the size and complexity of the RCC many commercially available clinical databases or computerised audit systems have used limited 'picking lists' to make the search through the RCC easier. The companies create these picking lists by asking the clinicians who will be involved with the particular computerised audit system to look through a list of Read Codes that pertain to their specialty and to select the ones that they are likely to use in the future.

For example, a general surgeon introducing a computerised audit system may be asked to check through the J Chapter (Digestive system diseases) and the section of Chapter 7 (Operative procedures) covering gastrointestinal surgical procedures. These selected Read Codes are then put into a separate table or picking list within the database. When the computerised audit system is operational this limited list is used as a first option to help locate diagnostic and operative codes for patient records, with the full Read Code list only accessible as a back-up.

Using a limited list has three main drawbacks. In the first place it is time consuming for the clinicians to have to search initially through all the Read Codes to select their limited list. In the second place it is constraining, because when the system is being used, if the most appropriate code is not in the limited list it is tempting for the coder either to choose the closest condition or not code the condition at all. (This sort of behaviour is most likely to affect the coding of important but relatively rare secondary diagnoses.) In the third place, limited lists are not usually updated as regularly as the Read Codes themselves.

The NHS Centre for Coding and Classification sends out regular updates to users via CAMS. These updates contain any new codes that have been added to the RCC database. However, many companies' computerised audit systems do not provide a way either for these updates to be added automatically into the full Read Code database, or for these new codes to be reviewed by clinical staff using the system so that they can be added to the limited list if appropriate.

Overcoming the difficulties

In spite of all these problems the Read Code probably still remains the best coding system for use within a computerised audit system. The NHS Centre for Coding and Classification itself is working hard on trying to overcome many of the difficulties outlined above. For example, to help resolve the problem of providing relevant codes in each specialty, in conjunction with the Royal Colleges the NHS Centre for Coding and Classification has set up a number of clinical specialty subgroups to advise on creating and maintenance of codes. As well as ensuring that the codes and terms used are optimal, the clinical specialty subgroups are working on the flagging of the codes within the RCC that they consider the most useful to their specialty.

In the past many of the problems associated with coding clinical data have been exacerbated by the practice of using clerical staff rather than clinical staff to perform the coding. If the input of clinicians is desirable in the classification stage of creating a clinical coding system, then the same is true when clinical codes are being used as part of a clinical database. Clinicians have a great deal of expert knowledge of clinical conditions, gained as an integral part of their training. Whether using the levels of the hierarchy of the Read Code database, or the RCC terms, keys, or synonyms, it is likely that clinicians are much more likely to be able to use the Read Code database structure correctly to identify the most appropriate Read Code in any situation. There are also many areas where the correct ranking of diagnoses as primary, secondary or tertiary can be crucial to maintaining the validity of the data.

For many reasons it is desirable that clinical coding is done by the clinicians themselves. These matters are discussed again in Chapter 12, but essentially the challenge that must be overcome by any provider of a computerised audit system is to develop a coding module within their system that encourages the clinicians to use the facility themselves.

Using codes to link clinical data

Up to now this chapter has covered the use of coded data to improve the accuracy of data entry and analysis, and the use of clinical coding systems.

However, codes can be used for a further essential function in a clinical database. Chapters 5 and 6 outlined the basics of relational databases. Recapping what has already been covered, in a computerised clinical relational database, all the details that are stored are stored in a number of *tables* which are linked together by *key fields*. For example, a patient's demographic details (name, address, date of birth and so on) will be held as a single record in a PATIENT table. At the start of each record there will be the patient's key field (patient identification number). When the patient is admitted to hospital on a particular occasion, details of the admission (such as dates of admission and discharge) will not be held in the PATIENT table but in an EPISODE table. Each record in the EPISODE table will have a unique episode key field, but each record will also contain the identification number of the patient to whom the episode belongs. In the same way, the clinical database may well have an INVESTIGATIONS table. Each result recorded will have a unique investigation number, and each result recorded in the database will also be linked to a particular patient, either indirectly through the patient's episode number, or directly through the patient's patient identification number.

It can be seen that the details of most of the data items which are stored in a particular patient's record are stored as key fields or codes only. These key fields then point to the full data items held in a separate tables. In our example of registering a new patient onto a clinical database, the most essential code in the whole registration process is the unique code that must be assigned to the patient themselves on their first encounter with any clinical database. The issuing of a unique number to a patient on registration is not only a requirement of computerised clinical databases, because the manual records in any hospital for each patient have always had to have a unique number.

In general key fields or codes used in a clinical database can be divided into two types. Some key fields codes will only be used locally, and they can be therefore created in any way suitable for local need. Other key fields or codes should be defined in such as way as to be universally applicable.

The use of local codes to link data

There are many situations where codes are only applicable to a particular system. For example, in most clinical databases, the staff codes will not need to be exported to any other system. These codes can therefore be allocated on an incremental basis, or they may be created by using the staff member's initials. Locally used codes such as staff codes can even be created by using the facility within the Read Code to create local codes within the @ Chapter. Whether or not these staff codes are created within the RCC, they only need to be comprehensible to the people using the particular computer system.

The use of universal codes to link data

There are many situations in a clinical database where it is useful or essential to create codes that can be used as a common currency across a number of systems.

For example, the RCC for diseases and treatments can only be used as a common currency if the codes themselves are centrally defined. In a similar fashion, the importance of using patient identification numbers to link all the information held about patients on a single computerised audit system has already been discussed.

Just like information on diseases and treatments contained within the RCC, patient data is also often held on a number of different clinical databases. In any health care system there is often the requirement to collate information on particular patients from a number of different sources. Even when these sources are computerised, this linking of information is usually frustrated by the lack of a common currency such as universally applicable unique patient identification numbers.

The importance of unique patient identification numbers

The concept of a unique patient identification number allocated at birth which follows an individual throughout their life carries with it suggestions of a loss of civil liberties, and associations with the idea of a 'police state'. In spite of this negative aura, it must be stressed that creating a common patient identification number would provide a number of benefits for both patients and the Health Service. At present many areas in the UK are now running centralised computerised cervical smear and immunisation registers, while at the same time the local hospital GP clerical staff are putting a lot of time and effort into computerising their records. Often the same information on individuals is held more or less correctly on a number of different clinical database systems even within a single area.

It is possible to link information held on different computer systems for the same patient by using a combination of non-unique data such as their surname, address and date of birth to try to match the records. However, such links are often frustrated by the fact that many of these data items do not remain constant. The same individual may change their name and address several times, even within the space of a few years. It is also dependent on the data being entered identically in each computer system, with no room for spelling mistakes.

In the next chapter the advantages of being able to link different databases containing clinical data within the same site will be discussed. A common patient identification number would greatly facilitate the passage of information from one system to another, so that much of the effort in computerising health records could be concentrated on recording the relevant, newly obtained information correctly rather than merely filling in old information already held on a computer elsewhere. At present the practical considerations of allocating unique patient identification numbers and enforcing their use on every encounter with the Health Service appear almost insurmountable. However, if the Health Service is ever to reap the full benefits of using computerised databases this problem will have to be resolved. The NHS Management Executive has recently decided that a new format NHS number will be created and introduced to act as a unique identifier throughout the NHS.

Summary

Any computerised system introduced for clinical audit will have a coded clinical database at its heart. This chapter has therefore discussed several important aspects of the use of coded data in a clinical database. The next and final chapter of the book will take up these themes along with many of the other topics already covered in previous chapters, and discuss how to design and implement a computerised audit system.

System development | 12

12

Outline

It has often been implied that audit can be done on the back of an envelope, and that the introduction of computer systems adds unnecessary complications to the process. This may indeed be true, but the contention of this book is that the introduction of computer systems can always aid the implementation of audit, and in some cases make the audit possible in the first place. It is vital to remember that the computer system chosen must reflect the overall aims and scope of the project. It is pointless to try to run a large departmental audit project on a single, rather elderly PC. On the other hand, it is equally pointless to insist that a small audit project cannot be attempted without the aid of a state of the art computer system.

This chapter outlines how to go about introducing a computer system for an audit project. It discusses some of the broader aspects of collecting and analysing data. As mentioned above, audit projects come in different shapes and sizes, so this chapter discusses the likely computer system requirements for three different types of audit projects. The first section covers the introduction of a computer system into a small audit project, such as an audit project run by a single enthusiastic practitioner in his or her spare time. The second section covers the introduction of a larger audit system into a department where it is likely both to involve the work of more than one practitioner, and to have to interface with the routine tasks of the department. The final section covers the introduction of a very large computer system which will cover several sites (possibly involving the work of more than one specialty), and in which the provision of data for medical audit is only part of the overall role of the system.

General considerations

Before going on to this detailed discussion, initial consideration of some general topics is required. The first concerns the overlap between the audit and management functions in any health care computer system. The second is the need to encourage conformity both in the use of data items and in the types of hardware and software employed.

Audit versus audit/management

Before installing a computer system for any audit project decisions have to be made about whether the system will be required solely to provide an audit function, or whether it will also have to provide non-audit management functions. Unpalatable as it might seem, unless additional resources can be found on a long-term basis, it is impossible to mount a large-scale computerised audit system that solely provides an audit function. The cost of installing the computer system initially, and the running costs in staff time, dictate that in many clinical situations the computer system will have to offer some advantages other than the ability to provide audit data for the clinicians alone.

In general, if the audit project it is to be a small affair completed over a limited time period, then it is likely that the work of the project can be done on top of the existing clinical work load. In this situation there will be no real need for the computerised audit system to provide management functions. However, if the project is going to be any larger or is expected to go on indefinitely, then it will have to pay its way – in other words it will have to provide some additional computerised non-audit functions.

These non-audit, management functions may be divided into two types: the first is that of providing paper-processing functions, the second is the provision of management information on the work of the department. The question therefore arises – if a computerised audit system has to provide management functions, what sort of management functions must it provide? Most clinicians would accept the proposal that a computerised audit system should provide paper-processing functions, such as the generation of discharge letters and routine clinical reports; and the management of a departmental workload by providing a booking service for tests and services. This is the automation of unrewarding and time consuming manual processes.

However, there is likely to be some resistance from clinicians when the issue of using a computerised audit system to provide audit information on the process and outcome of medical care to Health Service managers is discussed. Although there is probably a consensus among most clinicians that managers are entitled to some aggregated information on work loads and throughput, many clinicians are very wary of detailed and non-anonymised patient information being passed from a computerised audit system to anyone outwith their clinical discipline.

How this matter of passing patient data on process and outcome between clinicians and managers will finally be resolved will depend greatly on the shape the NHS itself takes on over the next few years. The introduction of NHS Trusts undoubtedly forces clinicians and managers to work more closely together at a local level, and the development of this closer working relationship is bound to be facilitated by the passage of better information between the two sides. This is discussed again later in the chapter.

The need to ensure consistency

Another important area to consider before commencing a detailed discussion of computerised audit system requirements is the issue of ensuring conformity. When any sort of computerised project is contemplated, it is essential to ensure that consistency is maintained not only in the actual data capture and entry, but also for the physical hardware and software that the system will run on.

Ensuring the validity of coded data As discussed in Chapter 11, it is of crucial importance that everyone who is collecting and using the data is speaking the same language. In any Health Care information system, clinical or managerial, it is vital that any ambiguity in the terminology used must be minimised. If codes are to be used, everyone must be aware of which codes to use in each situation, and what they mean.

For example, if data on the type of admission is to be collected, than there must be strict definitions as to what constitutes a GP referral, or an emergency admission or a planned admission and so on. If clinical coding is to be done, then whoever is doing the coding must be able to code the data in a consistent and comprehensible fashion.

Ensuring hardware/software compatibility If data is to be exchanged electronically, hardware and software standards must be set. Even where data is collected on a number of computers, it is possible to exchange this data by linking the different computers together. Every link between different hardware and software systems creates a potential problem area. In large computer system developments different users and pre-existing computer systems will almost certainly have to be linked from the outset of the project. It is essential that stringent standards are set at the beginning as some types of computer hardware and software are almost completely incompatible. It is essential be aware of these types of problem when introducing a new system.

Bearing in mind the overall requirements and constraints discussed above, the next sections will discuss the requirements for different types of computerised audit systems. The first section outlines the system requirements for a small audit or research project, the second section discusses the system requirements for a larger audit project, and finally the third section covers the particular requirements for very large audit/management computer systems which link the work of several departments.

Small projects

This section outlines the requirements to introduce a small computer-based audit project. A small audit project will probably closely resemble a small research project. As already mentioned, the cost, the amount of data collected and the time span of the project are all likely to be fairly limited, so it is usually possible to do such a project on top of the existing work load. There is often no need to design the project to provide any paper-processing management functions, or any data for health care managers.

The data for such a project may well be collected, entered and analysed by a single person. In this sort of situation it is very likely that the principal auditor will be a single individual, probably armed with a PC, an off-the-shelf software package, and some help from a secretary and/or the audit facilitator. (In the following discussion the term 'auditor' will be used to mean the principal researcher or clinician involved in the audit.) For most small computerised audit systems, even when secretarial help is employed, the number of people involved in the project is likely to be small.

For any sort of audit project, small or large, to succeed, it is very important that the aims of the project are set out clearly at the start. In a small audit project these aims can probably be summarised as follows.

Aims for designing a small computer project

The points that follow are summarised in Table 12.1.

Table 12.1 Aims for designing a small computer project

1 The computerised audit system chosen must collect information that is useful for clinical audit
2 The data should be collected and entered by the appropriate personnel, in an appropriate manner
3 It should be as easy as possible to access the collected data for analysis and presentation
4 The computer system should run on suitable software and hardware
5 The choice of system should be influenced by any hardware and software support available locally
6 If other people are involved in implementing the project, their cooperation should be sought at an early stage.

Aim 1   Collect useful information

The most important part of any project is to consider what areas of clinical practice will be examined. The next stage is to make sure that relevant data will be collected. In general, in a small project, it is essential to concentrate on trying to answer a particular question, rather than collecting masses of data in the hope that some of it may eventually come in useful. In a small project the auditor can decide only to collect the data that is of interest to the project – in contrast to intermediate audit projects coupled onto management systems, where it will be necessary to collect a much wider range of data items.

The two golden rules for collecting data for a small project are first to collect the data that will answer the questions, and secondly to try to avoid having to collect data that will be difficult to obtain. In a small project resources may be limited and time may be of the essence. The collection of prospective data is generally easier than the collection of retrospective data but in a small project it may be easier to collect retrospective data from clinical notes.

Aim 2   Use appropriate personnel to collect and enter the data in an appropriate manner

Once a decision has been reached on what data is to be collected, the next stage is to consider how the data will be collected. Where data is being collected retrospectively, if the previous records are incomplete or ambiguous, data collection will be difficult. The greater the knowledge base of the person collecting the data, the more likely these problems can be minimised.

Collection and entry of data by the auditor In an individual project, collection and entry of the data by the auditor has several advantages. By definition, the auditor will be closely involved and will have a vested interest in entering accurate information. Also, if the auditor is collecting the source data, there are much less likely to be difficulties entering complicated data items such as diagnostic and operative information.

Data can be collected prospectively or retrospectively from the case notes. Data can then be entered on to the computer either immediately or from paper notes. In both situations the auditor is able to use specialised clinical knowledge, either by recording accurate information prospectively, or by using his or her skills to make up for deficiencies in the recorded information in the case notes. In general, if the data entry is done directly by the auditor there is less need for elaborate contingencies to maintain the validity of the data on entry. The auditor is more likely to pick up any omissions and inconsistencies in the paper records before the data is entered onto the computer.

Collection of data by the auditor, but entry by another Even in a small project it may not be possible for the auditor to enter the data directly onto the computer. The data may be put onto paper by the auditor, for entry by someone else. In these situations the auditor must ensure that the information is as complete and accurate as possible. This is particularly important with medically generated data such as diagnoses. This data must be presented in such a way that it is easy for the other party to enter it. With these precautions the data entered is likely to be as accurate as if the auditor had entered it themselves. However, it cannot be overstressed that the auditor must ensure that the helper is provided with full and legible records to enter, and not presented with scrawled and poorly completed forms to decipher and code.

Collection and entry of data by others In this situation where the data is collected and entered by others, even in a small project, there is great potential for the GIGO syndrome – Garbage In Garbage Out. If the data is collected in a standard manner, the completeness and the accuracy of the data can be maximised as long as three simple rules are followed. The first rule has already been covered – adequate guidance must be given to those collecting and entering the data. The second rule is that the data must be checked after entry by the auditor. The third rule is that acting as a helper should be in some way beneficial to the helper.

To expand on the second rule outlined above, in larger computerised audit projects where the data is likely to be used to produce standard reports such as discharge summaries, it is probable that non-trivial errors in the information will be noticed and corrected. In a small project this type of data validation may not happen. If the data is collected by overworked staff who see this as an extra duty on top of all their other work, there is a good chance that inaccurate data will be entered into the database. These inaccuracies will not be picked up unless the auditor concerned checks the data personally on a regular basis. Regular checking will also discourage helpers from leaving parts of the database blank, or even worse – having a guess.

The third rule follows on from this. If the helpers benefit in some way by entering the data, they have more interest in ensuring its accuracy: for example, it is helpful if the data collected can then be used as part of the requirements for training.

Aim 3   Ensure easy access to the collected data

The whole point of doing any audit project (large or small) is to extract useful information at the end of it. The importance of choosing the right data items at the start of the project has already been stressed – it is obviously impossible to analyse data that has not been collected in the first place. Having considered how data should be entered into the computerised audit system, it is also essential that some thought is given to the ways in which the data will be extracted.

One of the main failings of computerised databases is the inability to provide easy access to the data that has been collected. As already outlined in Chapter 6, small computer programs (usually known as *queries*) are required to access the data contained in the database. The programs to generate these queries are written in a particular way, usually different for each type of database. Each type of database has its own *query language*. The ease of writing these queries depends on the type of database used, the way that the particular application program has been designed, how user-friendly the enquiry language is and the skill of the individual writing the enquiry programs.

It is obvious that the ability to analyse the data at the end of the project will depend on the type of computer software chosen and the level of computer skills present in the auditor or whoever is helping them. These areas will be covered in more detail in the section on selecting computer hardware and software that follows. However it is worth reinforcing the point that although computerised databases can output data in the form of routine paperwork, in a small research/audit project this may not be worth the effort, because of the size and the short-term nature of such a project.

Aim 4   Use suitable software and hardware

In a small audit project, it is likely that the computer database itself will be designed from an off-the-shelf software package by the auditor or their helper(s) and the software program will be run on a stand-alone PC. The following discussion will be based upon this assumption. However, it may be necessary to obtain customised software from another source. This is very likely to happen in a situation where the software will be used by a number of users, or the audit program will have to perform management functions. The acquisition and use of such customised software is discussed in more detail in the second section of this chapter, covering the installation and implementation of larger computerised audit systems.

Selecting the right software   The core of any audit project will be the database. It will be used to collect and analyse the data. In software terms, the choice of database is the most important decision to be made in the whole project. There are several question to ask before making a choice of database. First, how powerful does the database need to be – can it be the computer equivalent of a simple card index with a new record for each patient episode (flat file) or is it necessary to link a number of patient episodes to a particular patient (relational) (Chapter 5). In general terms, for an auditor with little previous computer software experience and with no local programming expertise available, the simplest/most user-friendly database that can perform the task should be chosen.

With the simpler databases it is usually fairly easy to design the data structure of the database and the on-screen forms used to collect the information. Designing the queries that will output the information in the desired format once the data has been collected may be more problematic. Simple databases may not provide powerful tools (graphing or statistical facilities for example) for analysing the data. It may be important to ensure that the data can be output in a standard format (Chapter 9) so that the data can be the exported into more powerful programs.

The results of these types of analyses can then be incorporated into a final written report.

Selecting the right hardware The assumption has been made that the system used for this small project will be a stand-alone PC, possibly even a portable or notebook. It is likely that this PC may be purchased by the individual auditor with money from a small audit grant. If a completely new system is to be purchased, it is desirable that it should be as powerful as possible and that upgrade options should be available so that the system can remain usable for the foreseeable future.

In this situation it is possible to use any sort of computer, such as a non-IBM-compatible computer, although it is desirable to use a PC if there is any likelihood of having to transfer the data to other users or systems. This allows the user to take advantage of other application packages or hardware that colleagues may possess. The PC chosen should be based on a 386sx chip or above with as much hard disk space as possible (preferably at least 60 Mb) and as much RAM as possible (preferably 4 Mb). Increasing the capacity of the hard disk can be expensive, so do not assume that it may be cost-effective to do this in the future. It is usually much easier to add extra RAM, so it is possible to skimp a little on the amount of RAM installed initially, as long as the computer has expansion slots (or even better space on the motherboard) for additional RAM to be added later.

A VGA or Super VGA colour monitor is desirable, but if this is too expensive, a mono VDU can be purchased, as long as the computer itself has a VGA or Super VGA video card so that a colour monitor can be substituted in the future. It is not necessary to purchase an expensive printer (especially if there is access to a good one for the production of the final written report), so a simple dot matrix printer will do. As defined at the start of this section, a small audit project is likely to involve only one user, so there is little need to consider the implications of having to integrate the hardware and software chosen into other computer systems. As long as file transfer can be done (using a floppy disk for example), it is totally unnecessary to worry about linking the PC into a network.

Aim 5   Choose the system in relation to the software support available locally

For any small computerised audit project there is unlikely to be the finance (or need) to provide rapid and professional support for the computer system. Such a system is unlikely to hold data that is vital to the ongoing care of patients. So as long as the data is backed up to floppy disk or tape regularly there is no requirement to consider comprehensive maintenance contracts for either the software or the hardware. However, in general, it is sensible to try to choose software and hardware that a knowledgeable colleague or friend is also using, because help and advice that is locally based and free can be invaluable.

Aim 6   Seek the cooperation of others at an early stage

In a small computerised audit project, the same individual is likely to be the system designer and project manager. It is unlikely, however, that they will be able to do absolutely everything in the project by themselves. In particular, if others are to be used to enter and/or analyse the data, the auditor must consider their training needs and the effect on their work loads. If the database is designed and used by the main auditor, it is not necessary to tidy up the system with easy-to-understand menus, nor is it necessary to train others how to use it. But if others are to be involved in using the system, it is important to make the computer program as easy to use as possible, and to provide adequate training for whoever is entering the data.

If the person who enters the data has never used a computer before, it is unreasonable to assume that a 15-minute demonstration of the wonders of the system will provide sufficient training. Efforts must be made to give proper training appropriate to the individual's needs, and user documentation should be provided if at all possible. It is also important to consider the motivation of the helpers and the effects on their work loads. If junior staff are dragooned into a project, without properly considering how and when they will collect and enter the data, the senior staff introducing the audit will be rewarded with incomplete and incorrect data in return. If the senior staff show an interest in how their junior staff perform the data entry, and take the trouble to give them as much personal support as possible (and regularly check the data entered), they will undoubtedly reap the rewards of this extra investment. The time scale of the project is also worth considering. It is easier to maintain everybody's interest in a project both if it has a limited life span, and if those who help collect the data are there to see the final results.

Larger computer systems

This section outlines the requirements to set up a larger computerised audit system, within a department, for example. Typically the system will operate within a single hospital department consisting of a number of auditors and their junior and secretarial staff, or within a single general practice. The system may or may not be linked to other systems outwith the department or the general practice.

Aims for designing a larger computer system

The points that follow are summarised in Table 12.2.

Table 12.2   Aims for designing a large computer system

---

1 The system chosen must collect information that is useful for clinical audit
2 The system must be able to automate the production of at least some of the routine
   paperwork and statistics
3 The data should be collected and entered by the appropriate personnel, in an
   appropriate manner
4 It should be as easy as possible to access the collected data for analysis and
   presentation
5 The system should run on suitable software and hardware
6 The system should link to other systems if this is advantageous
7 All efforts must be made to ensure that the suppliers of the system have the level of
   expertise to deliver the system that they have promised
8 The cooperation of the other people involved in implementing the project should be
   sought at an early stage
9 Adequate training, support and data security must be provided by the system
10 A project manager should be provided to oversee the implementation
11 Consideration should be given to the appointment of temporary staff at all levels
   during the implementation period

Aim 1   Collect useful information

It has already been noted that with a small project it is best to concentrate on
trying to answer a particular question. If at the end of a small project it has not
been possible to answer the original question from the data collected, it is
always possible to repeat the exercise, bearing in mind the lessons already
learned. With a larger project, however, it is likely that once the system is
installed, it will be a major undertaking to alter the system substantially. It is
crucial therefore to choose the right balance of data items to collect at the start
of the project. By the right balance it is implied that it is as important to collect
the required data as it is *not* to collect unnecessary data. It must also be
remembered that substantially altering the amount and type of data items
collected not only entails the re-writing of the software, it also entails re-training
of their staff using the system and these are definitely not trivial tasks.

In a larger project, there is also more than the individual auditor's information
needs to satisfy. Larger projects require substantial investments, both in staff
time and equipment. Therefore auditors initiating the project may have to accept
that the information needs of other groups may also have to be provided for. In
this situation the ideal approach would be to bring together all the interested
parties, including the clinicians, Health Service managers, medical record
officers, practice managers and clerical staff, and allow them to decide together
what sort of data should be collected. In practice this process is difficult to
achieve, principally because in many areas of the Health Service there is often
no clear understanding of what the information needs are. Good commercial
software companies are well aware of the requirements to get the balance of

data items collected right first time and they put a great deal of effort into trying to identify the data items required at the beginning of a project.

Aim 2   Automate the production of some of the routine paperwork and statistics

One of the requirements that the non-clinical users of a larger computerised audit system may well expect is the ability to produce some of the routine paperwork. However, it is unlikely that the system will be able to cope with the automation of all the routine tasks done by the department. It is important only to expect the computer system to automate areas where it is appropriate for it to do so.

For example, in a general practice setting it is obviously advantageous for the computer system to produce routine prescriptions. However, the advantage of using the computer system to produce once-off prescriptions as well (building a complete description data record for each patient) may be outweighed by the loss of the practical advantage inherent in the GP being able to hand-write these prescriptions during the actual consultation with the patient. It is important to maximise the advantages of using the computer system for routine paperwork, but not to be overambitious and try to replace all the manual tasks with computerised wizardry.

The production of routine paperwork can be used to drive the audit process. This situation is highlighted in general practice where, as mentioned above, one of the first aims in the introduction of a computer system is to automate the production of repeat prescriptions. This process builds up a database of patient information and in particular identifies certain patient groups, such as medication-controlled diabetics and asthmatic patients, and thus creates an easily accessible register of particular patient groups which can then be used to audit the clinical care they receive.

Aim 3   Use appropriate personnel to collect and enter the data in an appropriate manner

Once a decision has been reached on the type of data to be collected, the next stage is to consider how the data will be collected. Unlike a small computerised audit project, in a larger project it is often not feasible to collect retrospective data, unless this has already been computerised.

The choice of how to enter the data in a larger project is also more limited because in nearly all circumstances it is not appropriate for data entry to be done by the auditors themselves. This is because the amount of data entry required is likely to be large and the most appropriate form of data entry will probably be to have the data collected by the auditor, but entered into the computer by another member of staff. It may be possible to have the data both collected and entered by non-auditors.

Collection of data by the auditor but entry by another In a larger project, both the increased amount of data collected, and the longer time scale over which the data is collected, make it impractical for the collection of data by the auditor to be substantially different from the way that he or she has collected data in the past. Therefore, particularly as far as clinically trained auditors are concerned, the mode of data collection is likely to remain the traditional method of either writing by hand in the clinical notes, or dictating letters and discharge summaries.

In the past most doctors have recorded clinical data in a fairly freehand way, usually including only the data items that are relevant, and adapting the order that the data is transcribed or dictated to their individual tastes. In fact, as far as medical secretaries and medical coders are concerned, doctors are notorious for recording only the data that they themselves think appropriate to record – often this information does not include a unambiguous main diagnosis. For accurate audit, and indeed for accurate data retrieval for any purpose, the auditor should ensure that the data collected on paper (or on tape) is as complete and accurate as possible. It is particularly important that diagnoses are presented in such a way that it is easy for the data processor to enter the information into the computer system.

Collection and entry of data by others Where the data is abstracted and entered by others, there is great potential for the GIGO syndrome. The important ways of preventing this have already been outlined earlier in the chapter but, to recap, it is essential first to give guidance to those collecting and entering the data, secondly to check the data personally after it has been entered, and finally to try to ensure that the individual collecting and entering the data has some interest in doing it accurately and carefully.

Aim 4   Ensure easy access to the collected data

The importance of considering, right at the start of the project, the way that the output information will be provided has already been discussed. For larger projects this is absolutely essential. In order to access any collected data in a database it is necessary to be able to use the database query language to write small computer query programs. The ease of writing these query programs is very dependent on the type of database used, and the way that it has been designed. As it is likely that the database will be provided by an outside company, it is very important that there is a set of standard reports initially available on the system which will retrieve the data items most commonly requested, as well as a facility for the provision of tailored, ad hoc reports that can be run easily by any member of staff. These will include the routinely generated paperwork such as repeat prescriptions or discharge letters. An example of additional reports which may be available include the printing of a list of patients discharged with a particular diagnosis within a specified time period from a particular ward, with the enquirer able to determine the particular diagnosis, the time period and the ward, and able to enter these variables in at the start of the procedure.

The ability to create new standard reports and ad hoc reports must always be available within the clinical setting. It is not appropriate to have to call on the services of outside software suppliers or consultants to generate these, as this creates a barrier between the clinician or auditor and their data. If it is not possible to identify and train a clinical member of staff in the query language of the database, this function must be provided by training a member of the computer or audit support staff available locally.

Aim 5   Use suitable software and hardware

In a small computerised audit system the auditor involved is likely to be able to control the choice and design of the computerised audit system. This is less likely to occur in the installation of a larger computerised audit system for several reasons, the most important of these being that larger systems are likely to be more complex multi-user systems. As such they cannot easily be designed from software bought off the shelf by busy amateurs, no matter how enthusiastic they are about the project.

Selecting the right software As already discussed, the choice of the actual database software is very important. This choice is particularly important in the rare cases where the software will be bought in as an off-the-shelf system and customised in-house.

If the entire computerised audit system is purchased from an outside supplier, the database software will be hidden from sight under the software *shell,* or user interface, that the software supplier will provide. In this situation, it is important to consider the capabilities of the user interface itself. Is it able to be tailored to the auditor's individual requirements? Can it be designed to collect and analyse the relevant data easily? How can the data be presented – for example, can the data in the database be easily graphed or incorporated in a document? In situations where all the tools provided by the software shell for analysing and presenting the data are not ideal, it is important to ensure that the raw data can be exported into more specialised software packages.

Most of the larger computer audit systems will be expected to produce word processed documentation (for example, clinic letters) as well as the standard reports from the database, so the adequacy and ease of use of the word processing facilities incorporated within the package must also be considered.

These points can only be answered by seeing the system in operation. However, when a computerised audit system is demonstrated, it is usually done by the suppliers of the software, and they will undoubtedly try to show their system off to its best advantage. This means that they will concentrate on showing the strengths of the system while trying to conceal any weaknesses.

They will also know their way round the system intimately and this will mask any difficulties in the user interface.

The best way to find out the strengths and weakness of any system is to ask another user, and to try to use their system to enter and extract your own data even if this can only be done in a limited way. It is important to consider the opinion of all the other users of the system, in particular those that do the actual entry and extraction of data. It is advisable, therefore, when reviewing a system, to try to ensure that a secretary or clerical assistant who actually uses the system is present, and to encourage that person to give their true opinion rather than the one they feel you would like to hear. This is obviously a counsel of perfection, and it is often not practical for enough potential users to spend as much time as is really ideal examining systems in detail before making a choice. However, a thorough review of all the systems available at the outset of any project can prevent very expensive mistakes being made.

Selecting the right hardware Any computerised audit system may start off as a single-user system and have to grow to take in additional demand. However, when it is deemed that the situation initially demands a multi-user facility, this must obviously be considered from the outset. The choice of hardware is much greater in multi-user systems than in single-user PC systems. In general the capabilities of a single-user PC system can extend from a slow machine with limited memory and a small hard disk able to run a limited amount of software to a fast machine with plenty of memory and a large hard disk able to run the latest in PC software. The differences between these two extremes are dwarfed when it comes to considering the range available when choosing a multi-user computerised audit system.

Assuming that a larger computerised audit system comprises a limited number of users (perhaps less than 16) within a single unit or general practice, such a multi-user system can be served from a PC running appropriate multi-user operating systems such as Unix, networked DOS or Windows. A larger computerised audit system will require a mini- or mainframe computer. This sort of system will be discussed in the third section of this chapter.

With the number of people involved and the requirement for technical assistance, auditors are unlikely to have an entirely free choice of the type of hardware provided. Very often the type of hardware purchased for larger computerised audit systems is determined by the type of software chosen. In spite of this it remains vitally important for the users of the system to ensure that the initial choice of certain hardware is made correctly.

The first point to consider is whether the hardware system chosen will provide sufficient capacity at the outset. In other words, will the hardware simultaneously support the required number of users, and will it do so without becoming so slow that the users will not use it? Very often in this situation the speed of the system and the number of users it can cope with is determined by the power of the computer (or computers) at the heart of the system. In general the power of the system is determined by the amount of money that is spent on the hardware.

The second point to consider is whether there is an easy upgrade path for the hardware. In other words, is it possible to increase the capacity of the original equipment to cope with additional users or new functions in the future by adding onto the existing hardware? Generally, the ease and expense of upgrading a system is dependent on whether the system is based on proprietary hardware, or whether it is an *open system*. An open system is one based upon industry standards that a number of different manufacturers adhere to. Such systems have the great advantage that they do not tie the user to one particular manufacturer.

The ideal hardware system for a multi-user computerised audit project would be an open system of sufficient capacity at the start, with a well-defined upgrade path. This means that the initial hardware provides an adequate base at the start of the project, and that it can be extended as the system grows. The purchasers of a computerised audit system can therefore protect their interests to a certain extent by ensuring that the system purchased runs on a widely used operating system (such as DOS or Unix) and that the software suppliers either allow a choice of hardware or guarantee that the system can be extended by adding on additional features and peripheral devices provided by other companies.

Aim 6   Link to other systems

One of the ideals to aim for in the installation of a new computerised audit system is to ensure that the new system can interface seamlessly with any existing computer system, and thus allow the ready passage of data between systems. For example, in a hospital there may already be a pre-existing computerised PAS (patient administration system) which collects demographic data on the patient (name, address, date of birth) as well as details of their GP and so on. There may also be computerised laboratory and investigative pathology systems. In the ideal situation, if data can be exchanged between the new computerised audit system and the pre-existing systems, then the computerised audit system can load up all the demographic data it requires on patients directly from the PAS, and all laboratory and pathology results can also be channelled directly from the laboratory systems. In return, when accurate clinical data on diagnoses, operative procedures and complications is entered into the computerised audit system, this information can be made available to the PAS, laboratory and pathology systems. The mix of different types of computer systems present in most hospitals often makes it a very complicated task to interface one to another because of incompatibilities between the various software, hardware and operating systems.

The ideal link between different computerised databases is a dynamic link, by means of which data updated in one system is automatically updated in the second. In practice this can be hard to achieve. It is easier to create links between the two different databases. Information in the other systems can be accessed as required by the computerised audit system.

Searching a database on another computer can take from a number of seconds to many minutes. For example, it may take 20–30 seconds to load a patient's details from one of the other computer systems. This time delay may be acceptable if this is done only once and the data is then stored in the computerised audit system. However, this means that this data is stored in a *frozen* state, that is, it will not be updated in line with what is happening in the other system. The alternative of accessing the data from the other system as required may well prove unacceptable if it means that it takes 20–30 seconds every time it is necessary. It also means that if the link to the other system is down (or broken) at any point, the user of the computerised audit system will not have access to necessary data.

In every situation where it is possible to link a number of computer systems, as well as asking whether this is actually possible, it is also necessary to ask whether it is practical. In some cases, if the system to be linked to is not updated regularly the data contained within it may not be worth accessing. There may be more accurate sources of this data available. In general, for most small to medium sized computerised audit systems, if the link is not going to be helpful and it is difficult to achieve, on a practical level, then it is probably not worth pursuing. It is also important to consider the probable life span of the system being linked to. If there is a strong possibility that this system will be replaced in the near future then it is not sensible to expend a lot of time and effort on a link that will become redundant.

Aim 7   Ensure the suppliers have sufficient resources

From the foregoing discussion, it is apparent that installing a small multi-user computerised audit system is not a task to be undertaken lightly. Unless the hospital or GP practice can rely on an exceptional level of in-house computer support, it will be necessary to buy in a ready-made computer system from outside. This purchase includes the acquisition of the expertise needed to design and install the system in the first instance. It is essential to remember that software suppliers are like any other suppliers, they all have to sell their product to stay in business. It is therefore vital to establish whether they are being economical with the truth in describing their system's capabilities and their own abilities to design and install it.

An important factor in deciding how to choose a supplier (as opposed to a product) is to consider the supplier's financial viability. The ideal supplier should be a large and financially secure company able to provide a wide range of technical expertise to design, build, implement and document a computerised audit system. However, very often the systems produced by such companies rely on fairly old-fashioned proprietary technology, and their systems are often prohibitively expensive. It is worth remembering that large companies can fold as well as small ones, and that it is often very difficult to support a system based on proprietary hardware and software if the original supplier is no longer in business.

The alternative, therefore, is a small company offering a more modern product running on open or non-proprietary hardware. The risks of purchasing a system from such a source can be minimised if the supplier provides full documentation and bases the product on standard database software so that it is possible for in-house computer staff (or even another software company), to support the product if the original supplier does go to the wall.

Another alternative available in some situations is to install software that is produced by the NHS at a national level. These systems are often free to NHS users. However, the departments that produce these national systems operate under strict financial constraints and are often understaffed. Although it is very unlikely that overall support for this software will ever disappear, in the short to medium term it may be that the level of support that can be offered on a day-to-day basis may be extremely limited. Such systems are usually inflexible and the incorporation of new features can be long delayed.

Aim 8   Ensure the cooperation of others

The importance of ensuring the cooperation of others has already been stressed, and it is probably fair to say that this requirement becomes more and more important as the projected size of the computerised audit system increases. Ensuring the cooperation of the individuals who will be working with the new system can be achieved in a number of ways.

Initial support can be enlisted by liaising with the potential users of the system from the very start of the project, and keeping them fully informed of developments. It is important to consider how the proposed computerised audit system is likely to affect the way that these potential users will go about their day-to-day duties in the future, and to provide them with as much support as possible during the introduction of the system.

Consider the effect on workloads It is essential to consider the effect that the introduction of the computerised audit system will have on the users' workloads. Most staff can accept an initial period of disruption, and additional work, during the start of the project. But no matter how enthusiastic they are about the computerised audit system, most individuals are unlikely to be happy about a continuing, long-term additional workload. The computerised audit system itself must therefore provide a trade-off in terms of either speeding up or simplifying a task previously done manually. The only viable alternative would be to provide additional staff on a long-term basis.

Siting of equipment On a practical level, in order to enlist the help of others it is essential to consider the siting of the proposed new equipment. As most of the data entry will be done on computer terminals, and most of the paper output produced by printers, it is important to provide enough terminals and printers for all the users. These should be sited in suitable locations, and on appropriate furniture.

It is also vital to ensure that the siting of the new equipment itself does not disrupt the functioning of the staff using it. Printers should be sited near enough to allow the production of letters and discharge summaries at ward office level. The requirements for the provision and siting of equipment mean that as well as purchasing suitable hardware and software it is also essential to consider the practicalities of each work situation, and ensure that everyone has access to the equipment that they need. As the clerical staff who will be entering the data will have used typewriters in the past, it may be necessary for access to a typewriter to be maintained. Even with the most extensive computerised audit system, at some point a typewriter will be required to type the odd letter or envelope, so space should be reserved for one. Also, adequate storage space, sound proofing and ventilation must be provided as computer equipment can generate a lot of heat and noise.

As well as considering the access to the computer equipment for data entry and the production of standard output such as letters and discharge summaries, there must be access to the computer equipment for data extraction. There will also be a need for terminals for staff training so that these tasks can be accomplished without disrupting the work of other staff. When the total size for the computerised audit system is considered at the start of the project, allowances must be made for adequate provision of computer terminals for data analysis and staff training.

Aim 9   Ensure adequate training, support and data security

One of the main barriers to the introduction of any new system, whether computerised or not, is the so called FUD factor – fear, unease and discomfort engendered in the potential users of the system. As outlined above, some of these negative feelings can be assuaged by encouraging the participation of these staff in the design of the system, keeping them well informed of developments, considering the effect on their workloads and ensuring that the siting of the new equipment does not overly disrupt their usual way of working.

Training and support   Two important factors to consider are the requirements for training and technical support. In both situations it is very likely that the outside companies providing the computerised audit system will provide the initial training and support. It is important that sufficient initial training is provided, both for the staff that will enter and extract the data, as well as for the in-house technical staff who will maintain the software and hardware. At the end of the training process the staff who will be using and maintaining the system should feel confident to do so.

Although a maintenance agreement must be drawn up to cover support for major problems, as well as the provision of updated software releases, and any necessary additional training, it may not be practical or affordable to expect the company to provide detailed on-going support once the initial installation of the system has been completed. In each area it is, therefore, desirable that at least one staff member is trained and available to offer first-line support to users. This individual should be able to turn to the company, when required, for further guidance. This facility should be incorporated in the maintenance agreement. The individual's role in supporting the computerised audit system should be taken into account when considering their overall workload. It may be necessary to offer two types of internal support staff for the users, for although it is possible for a non-technical member of staff to supply first-line software support, it is likely that hardware support (covering malfunctioning equipment such as computers and printers) will have to be provided by staff from the computer services department.

In any system, there will always be a requirement to train new users to the system. This means that there must be designated members of staff who can provide training and support to existing users, but who also have the time available to train these new users. It is helpful if the training equipment can either be provided in a separate location, or at a time when the system is not being fully used, as any training is best done away from the day-to-day work on the system.

Housekeeping and data security Adding new users and removing old ones is usually termed *housekeeping*. This also involves the clearing of redundant files, issuing of passwords and taking regular back-ups. The issue of data security has not been touched on in detail up to now, but it is unlikely that any commercially available multi-user computerised audit system will be installed without issuing passwords and user IDs. Their use ensures that unauthorised users cannot enter the system, as well as determining the functions that are available to each individual user (so that only certain 'super users' can gain access to alter the actual functioning of the system itself).

For any multi-user system, it is essential that at least one member of staff be able to perform all the housekeeping tasks on a regular basis. These include the issuing of new user IDs and passwords for new members of staff (and for existing members of staff who have come back from their holiday and have forgotten their passwords). It is also absolutely vital to ensure that, while all members of staff understand the importance of regularly backing up data, at least two members of staff are not only trained to do back-ups of the system, but that they are aware that the integrity of the entire computerised audit system depends on them performing this task regularly and correctly.

It is unreasonable to expect the local hardware support team (or indeed the software company itself) to perform miracles. When they have to come riding to the rescue to restore a system when some major disaster has trashed the computer's hard disk, they will not be able to perform this function at all unless the users in turn can supply them with a full and up-to-date back-up of the data.

Aim 10   A project manager should be provided

It can be seen from the discussion above that installing any multi-user computerised audit system, no matter how limited, involves a great deal of organisation and attention to detail. Even the most enthusiastic auditor will not be able to manage the implementation of such a system and discharge their daily duties effectively. For any project to succeed it is essential that there is someone available to manage the entire project. Their first priority must be to assess the requirements needed to set up the system, and then decide on a time scale for the project, in conjunction with local staff and with the outside suppliers. The project manager must also be available to monitor the project, to keep everyone informed, to troubleshoot, encourage and cajole all around them. The task of project manager must always be performed by an enthusiast for the system, as there will be many times when the combined weight of user resistance, technical problems and lack of resources would cause all but the most determined individual to wilt and seriously consider packing it all in.

Aim 11   Consider the appointment of temporary staff

The role of the project manager has been outlined above. If the project manager is to be an existing member of staff, then it is essential that their colleagues, both clinical and managerial, support them. In practical terms this means relieving them of some of their other duties, at least over the implementation period. It is unreasonable to assume that any computerised audit system can be implemented without some additional resources, particularly in the short term. It is important that this point is accepted by everyone involved in the project at the start or the whole endeavour is almost bound to fail.

If it is desirable that a project manager should either be appointed as an additional member of staff or, if someone is appointed from among existing staff, that they should be relieved of some of their other duties while the computerised audit system is being implemented, then the same considerations must apply to other members of staff involved in the implementation of the computerised audit system. Although resources may not always allow it, thought should also be given to the provision of additional staffing support at all levels during the installation of the system. Training of staff in any new system is bound to be time consuming. All staff who will be using the system will not only require training, but they also will require time to come up to speed when they start using the system.

It may be cost-effective, in the long term, to appoint temporary clerical, secretarial and technical staff to provide additional support over the implementation period. This might avoid a backlog of work in all departments as staff struggle to learn about the new system and cope with their normal workloads at the same time.

Very large computer systems

In the two previous sections the introduction of small and larger computerised audit systems has been discussed. The provision of these types of system is a relatively new development. Until very recently, the majority of computer systems installed in health care facilities were extremely large. The history of the introduction of these very large computer systems into the Health Service has not been a happy one. Most of the systems have been hospital-based, and they have usually been designed to run patient administration systems and/or to collect data for the hospital management. Very often the systems introduced were old fashioned and unwieldy, difficult to operate and liable to go down at the drop of a hat. Perhaps that is why, in the view of the medical, nursing and paramedical staff working in hospitals, it has often appeared that the introduction of computer systems into hospital practice has resulted in a lot of disruption, without any apparent benefit to their clinical practice, as the clinical information collected by these management systems has often been too incomplete and inaccurate for their use.

In contrast, the recent introduction of computer systems for audit has been led by the clinical staff, rather than by the hospital management. (In the following discussion the term clinical staff will be used to mean nursing, paramedical and medical staff.) Usually these systems have been small-scale implementations, often based around a single PC funded from sources outwith the hospital computer budget. Although these small computer systems have usually fulfilled the needs of the clinicians, as far as the hospital management has been concerned, the information collected by these systems has been too limited in scope to be of much use for hospital managers wishing to obtain an overall picture of clinical practice.

Up to now, as far as the introduction of computer systems is concerned, the situation has been fairly polarised with Health Service managers and computer service departments busy introducing large mainframes and minicomputers to run largely administrative tasks, while clinicians interested in clinical audit have concentrated on introducing small PC-based systems.

The importance of working together

The divisions in the types of computer system favoured by different groups within the Health Service are fading. Changes in the way the Health Service is being run, and the move towards requiring better information and increased accountability in all professions, has meant that over the past few years the interests of both Health Service management and the clinicians have begun to coincide. Increasingly both managers and clinicians have begun to see the need for better information systems. The best way to obtain better information systems is for all the professions to work together. For example, there is no doubt that large computerised audit systems are extremely expensive to install and maintain and therefore the introduction of such systems for clinical audit alone is not feasible. On the management side, there is also little point in Health Service management introducing expensive computerised management systems without ensuring a better quality of clinical data.

It is fair to say that up to now there has been a resistance among some clinicians to releasing any clinical audit data, no matter how innocuous, to anyone other than their close clinical colleagues. Although this book is not the place to argue the whys and wherefores of who should have access to the data obtained from the introduction of computer systems, there is no doubt that both clinicians and management need to collect better data about what is happening in the Health Service. It is also apparent that both clinicians and management have a lot to gain from joint computer systems that collect accurate and relevant data with the minimum of disruption to clinical practice, and with as little as possible duplication of data entry.

It is of benefit for all professions to work together to introduce large computer systems. For the clinician it is of supreme importance that such systems should be capable of providing adequate data for clinical audit. The aim of this book is to aid any auditor contemplating introducing a computer system for clinical audit no matter how large or small. When introducing a large computer system, clinical audit is often merely one part of the jigsaw. Any clinician involved in the design and implementation of a very large computer system should try to ensure from the outset that the system will incorporate the facilities that they require. The sections that follow will try to offer particular guidance to the auditor involved in the introduction of a large computer system.

The importance of recognising the pitfalls ahead

It cannot be overstressed that introducing large computer systems into the Health Service is a costly and complex affair, and there is great scope for ending up with an expensive Frankenstein of a system which eats resources and refuses to divulge accurate information in return. To try to ensure that any large-scale computer system that is purchased is optimal to both clinicians and management, hospitals contemplating introducing such systems in the past have commissioned voluminous Operational Requirements (ORs).

Very often these ORs have seemed to delay progress towards a working system as both purchasers and supplier became bogged down in a morass of minute technical details. In contrast, because of the emphasis on technical matters, it has often appeared that not enough thought was given in the OR to a detailed appraisal of what the users actually required the system to do.

The projects have a huge remit and the time scales often become very protracted. There are often long delays between users being initially consulted, and the final project being installed. The implementation itself becomes a logistical nightmare, having to incorporate designing the software, installing the software and hardware and the training of the personnel who will use the system, alongside coping with the numerous technical problems of linking the new system to the existing manual and computer systems.

These problems often seem to lead to the project becoming a top-down development controlled by a shadowy committee composed of individuals far removed from the day-to-day running of the service. Instead of the immediate control of a small-scale system where the control of the project lies largely in the hands of the users themselves, it often seems to those involved in such large-scale projects that they are trapped in a huge and impersonal process grinding slowly towards some indefinite and distant conclusion. Often when the much vaunted system finally goes 'live' it appears to be slow, out of date and unable to collect and analyse the required information.

Aims

To try to avoid this kind of nightmare occurring the following section offers some guidance for clinicians involved in introducing very large Health Service computer systems. The aims of introducing such systems are in essence similar to the aims for introducing a large computerised audit system, as already discussed previously. Due to the enhanced scale of a very large computer system, however, certain of the points discussed in the section on the aims of a larger computerised audit system need to be amplified.

In covering the first four recommendations made in the previous section about data collection and analysis, the following additional points must be made for very large systems. First, like all computerised audit systems the data collected in a very large computer system must be useful for clinical audit, but unlike the previous computerised audit systems discussed it is essential rather than desirable that detailed management information is also collected. Secondly it is also essential rather than desirable that the computer system provides many of the routine hospital paperwork functions. In a a hospital computer system these routine paperwork functions will include computerised functions that are not directly connected with collecting either audit or management information – activities such as straightforward word processing.

Thirdly, because a very large computer system requires such a wide range of data items to be collected, it is of paramount importance that the different types of data items are collected by the appropriate personnel. As before, it is probable that clerical staff will be available to collect most of the data required. However as both clinical and managerial staff will now rely heavily on the data collected, it is as essential to the Health Service managers as it is to the clinicians that the clinical information is accurate. For this reason, it is very important that the

Health Service managers as well as the clinicians understand the necessity for the clinical coding facilities of the system to be top rate.

Fourthly, in terms of data analysis, it is crucial that efforts are made to ensure that the data is easily accessible once it is collected, because the more complex the data collection and the greater the number of data items collected, the more thought must be given as to how this data can be accessed.

The requirements to ensure that the computer system provides excellent clinical coding and easy access to the data lead into the fifth and sixth aims (pp. 149–152 above), that the computer system must be based on suitable hardware and software, and that it must also link to other computer systems such as the PAS, laboratory computer systems and financial computer systems if present. The final choice of an appropriate computer system may largely be made by clinical and managerial staff involved in the project, but they must ensure that they in turn are able to rely on expert technical advisers who have a good understanding of the information needs of the users. In particular, as the requirement for the computer system to exchange data with other hospital computer systems is now no longer optional but essential, the need for good technical advice is even more acute. (As an aside it should be noted that the approach taken to link disparate large computer systems within a hospital usually consists of installing a centralised large mainframe which can draw data from the other smaller computer systems. It is important to be aware that this approach does not necessarily mean that information can be passed through this centralised computer from one clinically or laboratory-based computer system to another.)

In the past, because of the vast costs of installing very large computer systems, the contracts to supply these systems have invariably been placed with big well-known computer companies who are very unlikely to fall into the hands of the receiver. This practice continues, so whichever computer company is chosen to supply the hospital-wide computer system, the system is likely to continue to be supported in the future. However, as well as remaining solvent, to satisfy the seventh aim outlined in the previous section (p. 152), the computer company chosen has to have the required level of expertise in understanding the information needs of the Health Service.

Finally, in terms of the actual implementation of the computer system (aims 8 to 11 in the previous discussion on large computer systems, pp. 153–157), there is even more need to obtain the cooperation of all the staff involved in the project, to give them adequate training and support and to ensure that watertight security and data back-up procedures are provided by the computer system and always obeyed. In a very large computer system adequate technical back-up in case of computer breakdowns is even more critical than before because once such computer systems are running, they will supersede many of the manual information systems previously used. This means that not only will the computer system invariably hold vital patient data, but also that it will also provide the vast majority of the paper-based functions.

For all the reasons outlined above, the installation of a very large computer system will be a complex and time consuming affair. It is essential that a project manager be appointed and the individual chosen must be highly motivated with a strong technical grasp of the situation. The ideal project manager should not only have a good deal of experience with computer systems but should also understand the information needs of the Health Service and be fully aware of how the delivery of health care is managed.

As a final point, it must be stressed that although small and to a lesser extent larger computerised audit systems can run successfully in isolation from the other computer systems within a hospital site, the project manager of a very large computerised audit/management system can only be effective within the framework of an overall information technology strategy that covers the entire local health care system.

Summary

This chapter has concentrated on applying the information provided in previous chapters to the actual process of choosing and installing a computerised audit system. It has looked in particular at how an appropriate computer system for each clinical situation can be chosen, installed and operated. The advice given in this chapter has been based largely on personal experience, and it is hoped that the experiences of the authors can be used to good advantage by others who are contemplating following the same path.

This chapter also concludes the book. It only remains for the authors to wish their readers good luck in any audit or computer-based projects that they undertake.

Bibliography

We have listed here the books we found useful when doing the research for this book. We also drew upon numerous computer manuals and magazines which have not been listed for practical reasons of space.

Benson, Tim (1991) *Medical Informatics*, Longman, London.

Hughes, Jane and Humphrey, Charlotte (1990) *Medical Audit in General Practice – A Practical Guide to the Literature*, King's Fund Centre, London.

Irvine, Donald (1990) *Managing for Quality in General Practice*, King's Fund Centre, London.

Irvine, Donald and Irvine, Sally (1991) *Making Sense of Audit*, Radcliff Medical Press, Oxford.

Jamsa, Kris (1991) *DOS the New Complete Reference*, 3rd edn, Osborne McGraw Hill, Berkeley.

Moving to Audit – An Education Package for Hospital Doctors and General Practitioners (1992) Centre for Medical Education, Postgraduate Office, Ninewells Hospital and Medical School, Dundee (funded by National Health Service in Scotland).

Rigby, Michael, McBride, Anne and Shiels, Chris (1991) *Computers in Medical Audit*, 2nd edn, Royal Society of Medicine Services Ltd, London.

Shaw, Charles (1990) *Medical Audit – A Hospital Handbook*, 3rd edn, King's Fund Centre, London.

Smith, Richard (ed.) (1992) *Audit in Action*, British Medical Journal, London.

Understanding Computers – Computer Basics (1989) Time Life Books, New York

Glossary

alphanumeric	The alphabetic characters in upper and lower case, the numeric characters and other characters printed on the keys of the keyboard. See also **numeric**.
ALT key	ALT, short for Alternate, key on the keyboard. It is pressed in conjunction with other keys to give commands to the computer.
ALU	Arithmetic logic unit, the part of the central processing unit that does the text handling and number crunching.
AND	Logical function used with Boolean algebra to query databases. See also **OR** and **NOT**.
application package	A computer program for manipulating data: for instance, a spreadsheet.
ASCII	American Standard Code for Information Interchange. An internationally accepted code for representing each character with unique binary values. See also **byte**.
assembly language	A low level computer language, a series of mnemonics each representing one command.
AUTOEXEC.BAT	A special file that is used by DOS when starting, or booting, up.
back up	To make a second copy of files held on computer. The back-ups can be used in an emergency if the originals become corrupted.
backing store	The part of the computer where information is stored so that it can be retrieved at a later date: see **disks** and **tape**.
bar codes	A series of black and white lines that represent numbers. The bar codes can be read by the computer to save the user inputting the number.

batch processing	The computer processes data, or instructions, in batches without any intervention from the user. See also **interactive processing**.
baud	A measure of the rate of transmission of bits from one computer to another or from a computer to a printer or modem: for example, 9600 bauds is approximately 9600 bits per second.
binary	The system using base 2 which has only two characters 1 and 0.
binary digit	A single digit that can be either 1 or 0.
BIOS	Basic Input/Output System; some of the instructions that are held in ROM.
bit	A shortened version of the words BInary digiT.
Boolean algebra	A type of algebra that is used with binary systems.
booting up	The process of starting the computer when it is switched on so that it can be used.
buffer	A area of temporary storage
bug	An error in a computer program.
bulletin boards	Areas of storage that can be accessed from many different computers.
bus	The wires which form the electronic pathway for bits to move from one part of the computer to another.
byte	A group of eight bits: see also **kilobyte** and **megabyte**.
cache	An area of storage which can be used to access data very rapidly.
Caps Lock	A key that causes each key press to produce a capital letter. There is generally a light on the keyboard to indicate that this function is on.
cathode ray tube	A tube, like those found in televisions, that is used to produce computer monitors.
CD-ROM	A compact disk that can store a large amount of unchanging information (Read Only Memory).
cell	A box on a spreadsheet.
central processing unit (CPU)	The heart of the computer where all operations are carried out: see also **chip**.
character	An individual number, letter or symbol. See also **numeric** and **alphanumeric**.
chip	The microprocessor at the heart of the computer.
clipboard	An area of intermediate storage where information from one applications package may be

	stored so that it can be used by other packages.
code	A fixed sequence of symbols to represent an object or concept. See also **Read Codes, OPCS 4** and **ICD9**.
communication software	Instructions that allow one computer to communicate with another.
compiler	A program that translates the instructions written in a high level language to machine language so that they can be executed.
computer	The central processing unit and other peripheral equipment that can electronically process data according to a set of instructions.
CONFIG.SYS	A special file that is used by DOS in the starting, or booting, up procedure.
control unit	Part of the CPU used to control the flow of information to the ALU.
conventional memory	The computer's primary memory where DOS and programs typically reside. Depending on the age of the computer it will be between 64 and 640 kilobytes
copy protected	A means of making sure that a program cannot be copied.
CPU	See central processing unit.
CTRL key	CTRL, short for Control key on the keyboard. It is pressed in conjunction with other keys to give commands to the computer.
crash	What happens when a program or the computer stops working.
cursor	The position on screen where the computer will show the next character. It is generally indicated by a flashing shape.
cursor keys	The keys with arrows printed on them. They control the movement of the cursor around the screen.
daisy wheel printer	A printer that contains a wheel with many spokes, with one character at the end of each spoke.
data	The information that is entered into the computer to be processed.
database	A type of applications package that can be used for the storage, retrieval and analysis of data. An electronic card index.
data types	There are a variety of different types of data that can be handled by computers. These

	include numeric (numbers), alphanumeric (a mixture of numbers and text) and graphic (pictures and graphs).
default	The value, or setting, that the computer will assume unless told otherwise.
desktop publisher (DTP)	A type of applications package that will allow electronic typesetting and page layout.
device	An electronic machine connected to the computer.
device drivers	Small programs that are used to give the computer instructions so that it can use the different hardware devices, such as a printer or a mouse.
digitisers	A type of input device. A magnetic pad that allows images to be handled by the computer.
directory	A grouping of related files that are stored on a disk.
directory commands	Commands that are used when handling directories on a disk. They are: CD for Change Directory, MD for Make Directory and RD for Remove Directory.
disk	A magnetic or optical medium for storing information that can be retrieved at a later date.
disk drive	The mechanism that rotates a floppy or hard disk, controlling its movements so that information can be retrieved from it.
disk heads	The part of the computer that will read the information from the disk.
DOS	Disk Operating System.
DOS commands	A series of commands that make up the operating system DOS. These are issued to the computer so that it can perform a specified task.
DOSSHELL	A specified DOS command. The shell produces a relatively user-friendly interface for using DOS.
dot matrix printer	A type of printer that produces each character from a series of pins. Each character is made of a number of dots.
double density	A measure of how much information a floppy disk can hold. See also **high density**.
down time	Time that the computer is not working due to a fault.
dump	To copy the contents of the screen, or a file, to either a printer or a disk.

editor	A simple word processing program that allows changes to be made to files.
electronic mail	Mail that can be sent between different users across computer networks. See also **bulletin board**.
Enter/Return key	The key, usually with a bent arrow drawn upon it, that is pressed to enter an instruction.
ESC key	ESC, short for Escape, is a key whose actions will depend on the particular application, but it usually takes you one stage back in a series of commands.
execute	To run a program.
expanded memory	A technique that combines hardware (memory chips and boards) and software (known as extended memory manager) to expand memory. See also **extended, conventional** and **higher memory**.
expert system	A computer program that is made up from a series of rules that can be used to aid decision-making.
exporting	Taking data from one application package and preparing it for use in another package.
extended memory	Combines hardware (memory boards) and software (a program called HIMEM.SYS which prevents different programs from using the same part of the memory) to make use of the memory, above 1 Mb. It is much faster than using expanded memory. See also **expanded, conventional** and **higher memory**.
field	A category of data. The information stored in a database is composed of a number of different fields.
file	The basic unit of information. A file can contain data or programs.
file allocation table	The contents page of a directory which gives a list of the files that are present.
file commands	Commands that are used when handling files on a disk. They are TYPE, to see the contents of a file; DEL, to delete a file; REN, to rename a file; and COPY, to make a copy of a file.
floppy disk	A removable magnetic disk, in a plastic protective jacket. They are generally $5\frac{1}{4}$ or $3\frac{1}{2}$ inches in diameter.
font	A typeface that can be produced by a printer.

font cartridge	A cartridge that can be plugged in to some printers to extend the number of fonts available.
format	A command which lays down the magnetic tracks and sectors on a disk or a technique which determines the layout of data within an application package, such as the paragraph formation within a word processed document.
freeware	Software that is available free of charge.
function keys	They keys labelled F1 to F10 (F12) either down the side or along the top of the keyboard. The actions of these keys can be programmed so that they can be used to give instructions to the computer.
games	A type of software that allows you to play games with the computer. The first commonly used ones were space invaders.
garbage in garbage out (GIGO)	The computer is only as good as the information collected. If the data input is unreliable the answers coming from the computer will be useless.
gas plasma screen	A type of screen used for some laptop computers.
gateway	Hardware and/or software that allows computers, on different networks, to communicate.
3GL	Third generation languages. These are the conventional computer languages like COBOL, FORTRAN, BASIC and PASCAL.
4GL	Fourth generation languages. These are a series of newer languages that are more similar to natural language so that even those with no computer experience should able to use them.
graphical user interface	A pictorial way to communicate with the computer. These types of interfaces are generally easier to use.
graphics	Production of pictures and graphs (non textual) using the computer.
hard copy	Anything that is printed out from a computer.
hard disk	A non-removable disk, usually sited within the main system box of the computer.
hardware	The physical parts of the computer.
Help	A system of assistance offered by most software packages where information about the package can be shown on the screen, often at the press of a single key (usually F1). Leaving the Help

	screen will return the user to the point at which Help was requested. Context sensitive Help will provide Help screens for the specific function being performed at the time of the request.
Heuristic	A rule of thumb, or method for problem-solving, that an expert has developed over years of practice.
high density	A measure of how much information a floppy disk can hold. See also **double density**.
higher or reserved memory	The area of memory between the conventional memory and 1 Mb. Part of it is reserved for interface to the video display and ROM-BIOS. This generally leaves a portion of 384 Kb unused. See also **conventional memory**.
IBM-compatible PC	A computer that has been designed to copy the original IBM PC. This means that programs written for the original machines can also be used on the compatible ones.
ICD9	International Classification of Disease 9th Edition. A coding system.
icons	Pictures that are shown on screen when using a graphical user interface.
index	Like an index for a book, these can be used with databases so that information can be retrieved more rapidly. See also **key field**.
ink jet printer	A type of printer with a cartridge of ink that is fired on to the paper as it prints.
input	A method for getting data into the computer so that it can be processed.
install	Setting up hardware or software for use.
interactive processing	Using the computer to have a dialogue with it. The computer responds to the user, one stage at a time. See also **batch processing**.
IT	Information Technology, technology that involves the use of computers.
I/O	Input/Output.
justified	A type of paragraph formatting, whereby the text is lined up along the left and right margins, as in a book.
kilobyte (Kb)	One thousand bytes. See also **byte**.
keyboard	An input device containing keys that allows the user to communicate with the computer.
key field	The field, or fields, that make up the index in a database. See also **index**.

LAN	Local area network, a way of linking micro-computers together over a restricted distance.
laptop	A small, portable microcomputer.
laser printer	A type of printer that uses a laser to form the required image on a piece of paper.
light pen	A type of input device that allows the user to shine a pen at the computer screen.
linear storage	Storing information on a tape so that it can only be accessed by playing the tape until the appropriate place is reached. See also **random access storage**.
line printer	A type of printer that prints each line as a single unit.
linking fields	Connecting one data base table to another. This is done by telling the computer that the linking fields represent the same data in the different tables.
liquid crystal display (LCD)	A type of screen used in some portable computers. Seen commonly in calculators and watches.
login/logout	Entering into a computer system or formally exiting a computer system. Generally used with multi-user systems.
machine code	A very low level computer language, communicating with the computer in binary.
macro	A small program, or series of instructions, that can be called by name and which will then perform the instructions automatically.
mail merge	The production of a large number of individualised letters from a standard template which is merged with a list of suitable names and addresses and other required information.
mainframe computer	A large computer that allows many users to use it simultaneously, often used for large processes such as hospital-wide systems. See also **microcomputer** and **minicomputer**.
megabyte (Mb)	One million bytes. See also **byte**
memory	Part of the CPU. Composed of the Read Only Memory and Random Access Memory. See also **ROM** and **RAM**.
Menu	A list of commands that will depend on the type of application program that is being used.
microcomputer	A desktop, or smaller, computer. See also **minicomputer** and **mainframe computer**.
microprocessor	The chip at the heart of the computer.

minicomputer	A medium sized computer, often running a departmental system. See also **microcomputer** and **mainframe computer**.
modem	A MOdulator DEModulator, used to allow computers to communicate with one another across telephone lines.
monitor (VDU)	The screen used as an output device for most computers.
motherboard	The board which houses the CPU within the computer.
mouse	An input device which can be rolled across a flat surface and causes a pointer to move on the screen.
multi-media	A new development where sound and vision can be incorporated into the use of the computer.
multi-tasking	The process whereby one user can get the computer to do more than one thing at once, for instance use both a spreadsheet and word processor at the same time.
multi-user	The process whereby more than one user can use the computer at the same time.
network	A number of computers connected together to share hardware and information. See also **LAN** and **WAN**.
NLQ	Near Letter Quality. Used to describe some printers that produce reasonable quality print out that can be used for correspondence.
normalisation	The process of building database tables, in a relational database system, that will optimise the performance of the database.
NOT	Logical function used with Boolean algebra to query databases. See also **OR** and **AND**.
Num Lock	A key that toggles the cursor keys so that they can be used alternatively between producing numbers or moving the cursor. Generally a light indicator on the keyboard will show whether the number function is on or off.
Open Systems: OSI	Open Systems Interconnection.. Standards being developed to enable different computer systems to talk to one another.
operating system	Software that controls the inputs and outputs of the computer and acts as a translator between the user and the computer.

optical character reader (OCR)	An input device that can scan printed pages and recognise the characters, thus saving the need to retype them into a computer.
optical mark reader (OMR)	An input device that can scan specially designed forms and recognise where particular entries have been made. These are widely used to mark multiple choice question papers automatically.
OPCS4	Office of Population Censuses and Surveys 4th edition. A coding system.
OR	Logical function used with Boolean algebra to query databases. See also **AND** and **NOT**.
output	A method for looking at the results of an operation that the computer has performed.
package	A piece of software or application.
parallel	A method of communication between a computer and other peripheral devices. The bits travel as if along an eight-lane motorway, in parallel with each other. See also **serial**.
parameters	Qualifiers that inform the computer of the object of a particular command.
parse	The process where the computer reads the data that is to be used by the application program.
PC	Personal computer.
peripherals	Hardware devices that are connected to the computer by a cable.
picture	This can be an icon on the computer screen, or other pictures produced using graphical packages. Alternatively it can be a pattern that the computer has to overlay on top of any data entered, when using a spreadsheet or database.
pixel	A picture element, the individual dots which form part of the picture the computer generates on screen.
plotter	A type of output device that can be used to plot intricate designs, traces etc.
pointer	A pointing device on screen which is coupled to the movement of a mouse. The pointer can assume a number of different shapes depending on the application package and its position on screen.
ports	Sockets at the back of the machine that allow peripherals to be plugged in.
printer	An output device that can be used to produce hard copy.

program	A list of instructions telling the computer what to do.
prompt	A series of letters that precede the cursor on the screen. These can say anything at all but it is most helpful for them to indicate the current disk drive and directory. For example C:\\>
protected mode	A way of using the computer so that programs can reside in extended memory. See also **real mode**.
pulldown menu	A menu option shown as one word on the screen. Once activated the choices available are shown as a list that pulls down from the original word. These menu systems are becoming more common especially in the more user-friendly packages including those that use a graphical user interface. See **WIMP, graphical user interface**
punched cards	An old form of input device. Each card had holes punched out of it and represented a line in a program.
querying	The process of asking questions of a database. See also **reporting**.
RAM	Random Access Memory. The working part of the computer's memory. The instructions to make the computer behave as a database or spreadsheet etc. are held here. Any files being created by the user are also held here. The memory is volatile. If the power is cut off the contents of the memory are lost. See also **ROM**.
RAM drive	Electronic disk drive. Data can be stored in the fast electronic memory and is very much faster to access than that stored in a mechanical disk drive. The information is lost when the machine is switched off.
random access storage	A method of storage whereby the average time to find any item of data will be the same irrespective of where the data is stored. These devices are disks. See also **linear storage devices**
Read Codes	The Read System of Coding for the classification of disease and treatments.
read/write heads	The heads that read information from, or write information to hard and floppy disks.

real mode	A way of using the computer where programs reside in memory below 1 Mb. See also **protected mode**.
record	A record is a row in a database table. It represents the set of data held about an individual or event, within the table.
reporting	The process of obtaining data from a database. See also **querying**.
robot	An output device that moves on the instructions of a computer.
ROM	Read Only Memory. Part of the computer's memory that holds the instructions required to allow the computer to boot up when switched on.
ROM-BIOS	ROM Basic Input/Output System. The program that loads the operating system and allows the computer to communicate to the peripherals.
root directory	The root directory is the top of the directory tree hierarchy.
scanner	An input device that can be used to scan images that can be input into the computer.
screen saver	A program that becomes operational if the keyboard, or mouse, is not touched for a pre-determined time. The programs either produce moving images on the screen which prevent a stationary image from being burned into the coating on the inside of the screen or turn the screen off. Touching any key will reinstate the original screen.
serial	A method of communication between a computer and other peripheral devices. The bits travel as if along a single-lane carriageway, one after the other. See also **parallel**.
shareware	Software that is available at very low cost, that the producers are keen for people to use and share. See also **freeware**.
Shift key	A key that is pressed at the same time as other keys to get the uppercase letter, or the upper character where more than one character is printed on the key.
software	The programs that instruct the machine so that it will process data.
speech input	A type of input where the user can talk to the computer.

spooler	A program that queues print tasks. A job sent to a printer is placed in a queue by the spooler until the printer is available. It is a mechanism whereby users can send several files to the printer at the same time.
spreadsheet	A type of application package that allows the user to manipulate numbers and perform 'what-if' analyses.
statistics packages	Application packages that allow the user to perform a variety of different statistical tests on the data.
system box	The part of the computer that houses the CPU. For most PCs it will also house the hard disk and floppy disk drives.
system disk	A floppy disk that contains some of the starting up instructions and DOS commands so that the computer can boot up. These are used on machines that do not have a hard disk.
tape	A form of storage device, useful for storing large amounts of data, where it will all be required to be read back into the computer at the same time. As it is a linear storage device it has limited use when used for small amounts of data.
tape streamer	A hardware device that allows the contents of a computer's hard disk to be backed up onto tape.
terminal	A screen and keyboard with no independent processing power. Used to communicate with a remote computer. Also referred to as a dumb terminal.
text	Information or data in the form of alphanumeric characters.
toggle	A switch which, when activated, alternates between a number of different conditions each time it is used.
toolbar	A region of the screen used by packages which have a graphical user interface. The toolbar contains a number of icons which can be used as a rapid way of instructing the computer without having to find the appropriate command on the menu system. See **WIMP, icon**.
touch screen	A type of device where the user can touch the screen to input information.

truth tables	A notation to explain the actions of the logical operators AND, OR and NOT in Boolean algebra.
TSR	Terminate and Stay Resident. Programs that can be loaded into the memory and remain there, even when not in use.
upper memory blocks (UMB)	A way of using reserved (higher or upper) memory, to allow data to be stored, that frees up the (lower) conventional memory.
user-friendly	Indicates that a piece of software is easy for novices to learn how to use. It is an often misused phrase.
utility	A program designed to make use of the computer easier.
validation	A method for checking data as it is entered to help ensure its accuracy.
virus	A type of program that can replicate itself and infect a machine. At some predetermined signal it can cause a variety of different, often damaging, effects.
WAN	Wide area network. A way of linking computers together over very large geographical areas. See also LAN.
wildcards	Characters that can be used to replace other characters, like jokers in a pack of playing cards.
WIMP	Windows, Icons, Mouse, Pulldown menus, the components of the user-friendly graphical user interfaces.
window	When using a graphical user interface, a window is part of the computer screen where the functions being performed can be seen. If several different functions are being performed at the same time each will have its own window. The user can jump between the windows. Windows is also the name of an applications package, produced by Microsoft.
word processor	A type of applications package that allows the user to manipulate text.
word wrap	The automatic production of a new line when typing, the words being automatically moved to the next line. This means that the user does not have to press the carriage return key as when using a typewriter.

write protect

A means of protecting a floppy disk so that no alterations can be made to the contents: no further data can be written to it.

WYSIWYG

What You See Is What You Get. Applications packages written for the graphical user interfaces often show the text on screen as it will appear on the printed page. This includes both layout and character formatting.

Index

Page numbers appearing in **bold** refer to figures and page numbers appearing in *italic* refer to tables.